Endorsements

"What a thorough, yet easy-to-understand and implement set of guidelines. Dr. Reinertsen empowers regular people across the globe to take their oral-systemic health into their own hands. His advice will not just change how you choose a dentist, but also how you view your mouth, and discuss your oral health with your medical providers. A shift is occurring and if you read this book you will be an important part of it!"

—Jamie Freitag-Dooley, RDH, BIS

Oral-Systemic Thought Leader & Founder of National Network of Healthcare Hygienists

"There is no shortage of passion from Dr. Chuck as he reveals the connection between your mouth and your overall health. From practical tips and tricks that you can do at home to expert guidance addressing other medical issues, this book is eye-opening and sure to be a great addition to your collection."

—Kelli Carter, MAADOM

"Are Your Teeth Making You Sick? is a helpful guide full of important information for those of us who wish to take the necessary and, oftentimes, overlooked steps toward better overall wellness. Having seen firsthand the effects that dental care, and lack thereof, can have on a person's health, this book particularly resonates with me. It's the wake-up call that some of us need to connect the dots between what should be obvious but, instead, goes commonly unmentioned in the medical profession. It just makes sense! My "why" is providing my little one with a healthy lifestyle and fully equipping him with all the tools he needs to be successful, including creating an effective oral homecare routine he can carry on into his adult years."

—Jaime Tewksbury, Dental Office Manager

"In my 20+ years of experience in the dental field, I was never trained on the connection of the mouth and the rest of the body until I had the pleasure to work with the author of this book, Dr. Charles Reinertsen. When he first explained the connection between the mouth and the rest of the body, it opened my eyes and showed me that the treatment of most common dental issues can solve many systemic diseases within the body. I witnessed firsthand his process with Alice, Debbie, and Melissa whom he was able to help, along with so many more who came through our door every day. I am so glad he decided to write this amazing book to continue his mission of educating the public about the connection between the mouth and the rest of the body. I firmly believe that overall health cannot be achieved without a healthy mouth."

—Marieta, Dental Assistant

"Great book! I wish I had this book years ago. Easy to read and understand. The author is very clear about what works and what doesn't work with dental care/oral hygiene. Now I can read this book with my daughter, show her illustrations, and explain more about our teeth. This book is a wonderful gift for families."

—Mira, Mother

ENDORSEMENTS

"Dr. Charles Reinertsen has written a must-read book about the long-ignored link between the mouth and the rest of your body. Read this book and regain control of your health."

—**Nelly R. Unger, DMD**

"My family has personally been affected by oral infections that have manifested in a major way in their bodies.

- My dad had a heart attack at age 43 and almost died. They found no blockages—only an infection in his mouth. This infection led to the attack.

- My brother John, at age 48, had elevated liver levels last summer. No cause could be found in the hospital—until they realized his wisdom tooth socket was deeply infected causing the liver to react.

I wish that my family had known this information earlier. It would have helped."

—**Deb, Patient**

"This book is outstanding. I can only imagine all the people this book will help to discover the real cause of their problems. Dr. Chuck's book addresses all three factors. How exciting to envision all the potential benefits this information could add to the quality of people's lives.

And to think this invaluable knowledge has been "right under my nose." This book should be required reading for all physicians."

—**Dr. Dennis Frerking, Chiropractor, Nutritionist, Lecturer**

"The discoveries of Dr. Reinertsen in his successful 40-year dental career will transform your thinking about the power in your mouth—power to give you a longer, healthy life—or power to breed illness leading to death. The wisdom found here changed my life!"

—**Doug, Patient**

ARE YOUR TEETH MAKING YOU SICK?

THE ANSWER IS RIGHT UNDER YOUR NOSE!

BY DR. CHARLES REINERTSEN

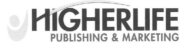

HIGHERLIFE
PUBLISHING & MARKETING

Special thanks to my editor, Esse Johnson, and illustrator, Mira Fallbeck

Are Your Teeth Making You Sick?

The Answer Is Right Under Your Nose!

© 2023 Charles Reinertsen

All rights reserved.

ISBN: 978-1-958211-14-4 paperback
ISBN: 978-1-958211-15-1 eBook

Library of Congress case no. 2023909147

Published by: HigherLife Development Services, Inc.
PO Box 623307
Oviedo, FL 32762
(407) 563-4806

www.ahigherlife.com

No part of this book may be reproduced without written permission from the publisher or copyright holder, nor may any part of this book be transmitted in any form or by any means electronic, mechanical, photocopying, recording, or other, without prior written permission from the publisher or copyright holder.

Printed in the United States of America

10 9 8 7 6 5 4 3 2 1

Dedicated to families everywhere.

INDEX

Introduction

Before you head into this book about oral health, you should know that this book is not strictly about oral health. It's about your body.

Once you've read the pages that follow, you will know exactly how to solve many dental concerns at home on your own. You will know how to shop for a great dentist and identify when you *really* need one. Perhaps more urgently, you will understand the relationship between your mouth and the rest of your body—a little thing called the "oral-systemic connection." This is the very real and vital connection between your mouth and every cell, muscle, fiber, organ, and tissue throughout the rest of your body.

For generations, ignorance of this connection has caused masses of people to needlessly suffer avoidable pain, sickness, and premature death. I hope that you will be the change in this silent epidemic, and that your success will inspire those around you to take the simple steps outlined in this book to prevent lifelong pain and possibly early death.

Don't read this book to find out how to get a Hollywood smile. Read this book to learn how to protect yourself and your family from harm. Take the steps herein to maintain lifelong health and well-being by taking good care of the one body part medical schools barely include in their education and physicians seldom check, but which is largely responsible for preventing disease and protecting your organs—your mouth.

A healthy mouth is one of five essential ingredients to your health.

1. Diet and medications: Know what you put into your body, both good and bad.

2. Exercise: You don't have to join the gym, but you do have to move and exercise daily.

3. Oral Health: Connect the dots between your mouth and every organ in your body.

4. Sleep: Your body does its best healing during sleep.

5. Attitude: Controls your entire life.

All five ingredients are necessary for a healthy body. For four out of five of these topics, hundreds of books have been written directly to families and non-medical people, but not many have been written on #3 explaining the medical reasons why your dental health is so important to your overall health. Many physicians will no doubt appreciate this book, but I've written it especially for the non-medical person to connect the dots between dental health and overall medical health. Once you "get it," you'll want to share it with your family, friends, and probably the medical professionals in your life, too.

You'll learn some surprising facts about tooth and gum infections.

You'll learn why it's not only possible but *likely* that you and your loved ones are carrying undetected infections in your mouth right now, which are depositing harmful, disease-causing bacteria into your body.

You'll learn why most physicians do not ask about your dental health.

You'll learn where dental bacteria go beyond the mouth and what they do to your body.

You'll learn steps you can take at home to help avoid serious concerns including cardiovascular, diabetic, pregnancy complications, and more.

You'll learn what you and your family can do to help avoid many health issues from bad breath all the way to death.

Soon, you'll see your mouth in a whole new light.

The next time you step into your bathroom and look into the mirror, realize that the source of many diseases is literally "right under your nose!"

Chapter 1

The Front Door to Your Body
The Invasion

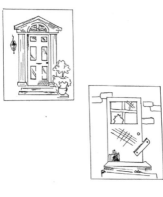

According to *The American Heritage Dictionary of the English Language,* an infection is an "invasion of bodily tissue by pathogenic microorganisms." That's a mouthful! Simply, this definition teaches us that an "infection" is also an "invasion." That is, before an infection can happen in the eyes, lungs, heart, brain, or any other body part, foreign invaders must somehow enter your body.

"I thought this book was about dental health?" you ask.

It is.

Every time you look in the mirror you are staring at a secret door to your body right there under your nose. Your mouth is more than a pretty smile. Your mouth is the front door to your body—and it's not just about what you swallow when you eat. The vulnerable spaces in this door can be both subtle and far more dangerous than you realize.

Allow me to share about Alice, Debbie, and Melissa. Their stories illustrate the astonishing, life-changing results you and your loved ones can experience by simply taking good care of the "front door" to your body.

Alice

Alice is an artist, but for two whole years, she had lost her desire to draw or do much of anything she enjoyed. On dialysis for several years, Alice was now bleeding excessively when nurses unhooked her from the dialysis machine. Her medications weren't working well. She had no energy. The only body part that didn't seem to experience daily pain was her mouth. At least her mouth was okay, right?

Then, one day, it happened. Alice finally got a toothache. She hadn't seen a dentist for years because nothing in her mouth had any pain. Her toothache drove her to find a dentist and I was the lucky dentist she found. It's a good thing, too, because that toothache was about to change, and possibly save, her life.

When I first met Alice, she looked rough. When she opened her mouth, she looked really rough. The bad news was that Alice didn't just have one infected tooth causing the pain. Her mouth was full of broken teeth and severe gum disease—a *dental disaster*. Think about all that breakage and gum infection like a tattered and rotting front door. With so much damage to her door, there was no telling how many invaders (bacteria) regularly passed through it into her body, nor how much of her suffering could be alleviated by fixing it.

That was the bad news. The good news was that the treatment was straightforward: get the infections under control with antibiotics and remove the bad teeth. By removing the infections and letting the gums heal, we effectively repaired and sealed (closed) the front door to Alice's bloodstream. After that, all that was left was to watch for improvements in Alice's health.

Within three weeks of treatment, Alice felt like a new person. Her excess bleeding was eliminated, her medications worked better, and her energy increased. Today, Alice has gone back to drawing and enjoys being alive again. Much of what she had lost is now restored—all by repairing and maintaining the front door to her body. Priceless!

The next story might be even more surprising.

Debbie

Debbie went to her physician with an abscess on her thigh. The doctor put her on antibiotics. The abscess disappeared for a few weeks and then re-appeared. The doctor put her on another round of antibiotics. The abscess again disappeared and again returned a few weeks later. After its third re-appearance, the doctor decided to culture the bacteria to identify it.

The results: dental bacteria.

Debbie hadn't seen a dentist for years because nothing in her mouth hurt. She had no pain, so she had no need to see a dentist, right? Nevertheless, the abscess on Debbie's leg was coming from harmful bacteria in her mouth.

During her first visit, we found three totally pain-free abscessed teeth. Debbie was shocked.

How can infections this severe not hurt? How can so much bone loss take place without any pain? That's the challenge. It's hard to believe, but it's true.

Three weeks after treating her abscessed teeth, Debbie's leg healed all on its own.

You read that right. We treated Debbie's dental abscesses—and her *LEG* healed. It's the other end of the body, yet it was infected by dental bacteria, and it was remedied by restoring her mouth.

Maybe dialysis or a leg abscess seem unlikely to you. How about something more common, like high blood pressure?

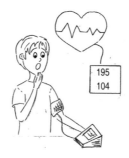

Blood pressure checking/ high blood pressure

Melissa

Melissa is a nurse. The only medication she was on was for high blood pressure. Her physician checked her blood pressure. It was high so they gave her pills to lower her blood pressure. Her blood pressure went down. Everything's okay, right?

When she came to see us as a new patient, we did an examination. We found a dental abscess. It didn't have any pain. She felt a little something, but not really any pain.

We took care of her abscess. In this case, we put her on antibiotics and then a few days later removed a hopeless tooth. She came back after about three weeks and said, "Guess what? I don't need my blood pressure medication anymore."

Can a dental infection raise your blood pressure? Absolutely! An infection anywhere in your body can raise your blood pressure. Your body is fighting the infection!

More often than you know, disease-causing bacteria are quietly entering the body and organs through damaged teeth, gums, or other tissues that make up the front door called your mouth and are damaging your body.

The River Inside You

If a factory polluted your drinking water, would you be concerned? ABSOLUTELY! Would you continue drinking it just because it tasted good? I hope not.

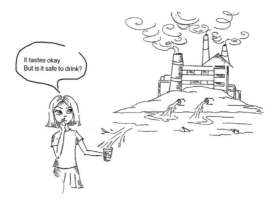

So long as you wanted to stay healthy and not poisoned by the factory's pollutants, you'd demand someone clean up that factory, especially if you had children drinking the same water.

We don't have a literal river in our bodies, but we do have a stream. It's called the bloodstream. Your mouth is the factory that can silently dump toxic waste pollutants into your bloodstream. There is no pain. There are no symptoms. You don't even know it's happening—but it is. Just like rivers, the bloodstream can become polluted.

What is the pollution? Let's follow the process.

Pus

Infections in your body produce pus. Anywhere you have an infection, be it from a scraped knee or a cut foot, you might have seen the whitish, creamy, smelly substance that oozes out of the wound—pus. Pus is comprised of harmful bacteria, dead tissue debris, dead white blood cells (WBCs), inflammatory proteins, and some other toxins. When the pus is external, like a pimple on your cheek, you can see it with your naked eye. It's an external infection because it's visible outside of your body. When you pop a pimple, the stuff that oozes out is pus. Because you can see an external infection, it's easy to clean, disinfect, and, if necessary, bandage the open wound.

When it's internal, such as an oral infection hidden behind the curtain of your lips, the pus is formed under your gums or inside the tooth or bone. From there, the pus can either drain into your mouth or into your bloodstream. If it drains into your mouth, you may notice a metallic taste, like sucking on a copper penny. Usually, there is no pain, but there is still destruction. If it drains into your bloodstream, the same is true only you never see or taste it. The pus goes from the infection into blood vessels located in your teeth, gums, and bones. Via those blood vessels, the pus travels past your front door and, thus, begins its journey through your body.

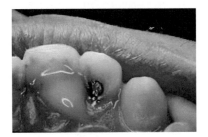

Carried through your bloodstream, this pus brings all of its dead cells and toxic waste through your veins to your heart; from your heart to your lungs; from the lungs back to your heart, which then pumps the infection throughout your entire body. This is the oral-systemic connection. Your mouth affects your whole body!

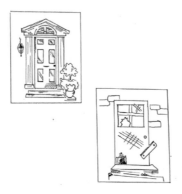

Imagine your mouth like a beautiful front door. Then, imagine it as a dirty, broken front door instead. How does that make you feel? One of these is true for you, but do you know which one? Ultimately, you won't know until someone skilled takes a thorough look.

Treat the Source, Cure the Problem

We use our mouth every day for talking, eating, and drinking, but do we ever consider it the possible source behind headaches, persistent coughs, or a stuffy nose? How about cardiovascular disease, heart attacks, strokes, pneumonia, E.D., diabetic and pregnancy complications, Alzheimer's disease, and rheumatoid arthritis?

It's bad enough that most people have no idea when their teeth are abscessed or their gums are infected. Even more devastating is the belief that oral infections only affect the teeth and gums. This is not true. Oral infections can cause or worsen many diseases throughout your entire body.

People frequently treat a medical condition for years without looking for the source. If you never eliminate the cause of the sickness, you will be on treatments for the rest of your life. Regrettably, much of our medical community today is quick to treat symptoms without even so much as looking for the source of the disease. That's the bad news. The good news is that if you can identify and eliminate the origin of the problem, you can dramatically diminish or even eliminate the diseases, sicknesses, injuries, inflammation, and overall unwellness caused by it—no further treatment required.

Remember Alice? She was suffering with excessive bleeding, ineffective medications, low energy, and overall depression. What was her treatment? Antibiotics killed her oral infections while tooth extractions removed the source. That is all. Once we cleaned up the factory and sealed it off from her bloodstream, her body could repair and heal itself. *No additional medications were needed.* That is what happens when you successfully identify and eliminate the source—in her case, a factory that was constantly dumping toxins in the river called her bloodstream. Once the factory was sealed off from the stream, she experienced dramatic healing and restoration.

You Don't Know What You Don't Know

If your teeth or gums don't hurt, they're healthy, right? WRONG!

This is one of the biggest hurdles we face when fighting dental disease. Most people believe that if there is no pain, their mouth is healthy. Usually, it's not.

Part of our challenge is limited visibility. It's dark in there. You have lips, a tongue, teeth, saliva, cheeks, and, to top it all off, a gag reflex. These can make it tough to conduct your dental self-examination. The dentist uses special lights and mirrors, not to mention X-ray machines. Doing that by yourself from home is not possible. If you do pull back your lips and look at your teeth and gums, do you know what you're looking for?

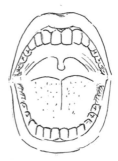
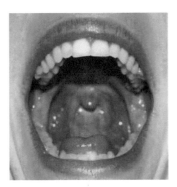

Do you know what you're looking for?

Even your dentist relies on a thorough clinical exam to see that your mouth is healthy. At a minimum, a thorough examination must include multiple radiographs (X-rays) to see beyond the surface. In forty-plus years as a dentist with my own practice, we rarely examined a new patient who wasn't suffering from a symptom-free dental infection. It is a fact that dental infections *usually* have no pain and, yes, *most* of my new patients were already carrying pain-free dental infections ranging from mild gingivitis to severe tooth abscesses with significant bone loss.

What's more, a patient's painless oral condition could be secretly linked to other symptoms that *are* painful such as headaches, lesions, swollen ankles, and joint discomfort. It's hard to believe, but it's true. When you consider that high blood pressure doesn't hurt and neither does diabetes, glaucoma, or cancer until the end stages, it's easier to understand that dental infections don't have to hurt to be damaging your body.

Can Dental Infections Really Be Pain-Free?

When you consider that neither high blood pressure nor type 2 diabetes cause pain, or that glaucoma or cancer can go virtually symptom-free until the end stages, does it become easier to accept that dental infections don't have to hurt to be damaging or even life-threatening?

Like so many, Alice saw physicians on a regular basis for years; yet, none of them picked up on her dental disease. Often, the source of a medical problem isn't really hidden. We're just not looking in the right place. Physicians weren't trained to examine your mouth. Most still seem to believe the mouth is only of concern to dentists despite the effect oral health has on the systems and organs of the body. Debbie, Alice, and Melissa had health problems outside of their mouths, yet the mouth was the source.

So, what do you think? Maybe we shouldn't consider our yearly check-up complete until we've thoroughly assessed the health of the mouth. Before assuming we have all the information to determine the source of a disease, we might do well to call in the dentist. You don't have to wait for your physician to ask. In fact, you probably shouldn't. As we'll unpack in the next chapter, waiting for your physician to ask for a dentist's oral report could leave you waiting a long, long time.

You'll need to see a professional dentist at some point, I'll show you how to get started at home, on your own, for less than two tickets to a movie theater (and maybe less than the popcorn). I've helped a lot of people rebuild and maintain a beautiful, strong, secure front door to their body and, through this book, I am grateful for the privilege and opportunity to show you how also.

Let's review what we've learned so far:

1. The mouth is the front door to the body. Most bacteria enter the body through the front door. These bacteria cause or affect many medical problems: cardiovascular disease, heart attacks, strokes, E.D., diabetic and pregnancy complications, pneumonia, Alzheimer's disease, and rheumatoid arthritis. Lack of pain does not mean the mouth is healthy.

Chapter 2

Why Most Physicians Are in the Dark about Your Mouth

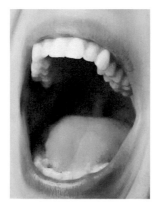

Over the last several years, I've asked my patients, "When was the last time your physician asked about your mouth?"

Usually, the response is, "Never."

How about you? Has your physician *ever* asked about your dental health?

Is Your Mouth Part Of Your Body?

If you've undergone heart surgery, your cardiologist may have requested a "Dental Clearance" from your dentist. Cardiologists know that if you're carrying undetected dental infections during heart surgery, the chances of life-threatening complications dramatically increase. Dental Clearance tells the cardiologist that you don't have an oral infection leaking bacteria into the bloodstream and potentially leading to major surgical complications. Cardiologists routinely request a Dental Clearance, but what about all the other surgeries with the same potential for disaster in the presence of mouth infections?

Occasionally, I've heard of a doctor asking when the patient last visited their dentist, but the inquiry stops there. In over 40 years of practice, never once has a physician requested I provide a dental health report as part of their patient's overall health assessment or treatment plan.

The standard medical "complete" physical examination does not include the mouth. Physicians have been trained to believe that the dentist has the mouth covered, so it's not their territory. Physicians are simply doing what they were trained to do.

They are correct that dentists have the structures in the mouth covered but what we don't have covered is the bloodstream. Infections in the mouth deposit bacteria into the bloodstream—the physician's terrain. Once in the bloodstream, bacteria hitch a ride to anywhere and everywhere your blood travels, reaching vital organs and tissues and compromising your health. This is why the mouth-body connection necessitates dentist-physician communication, even if it's the patient (you) who must bridge the deadly gap between them.

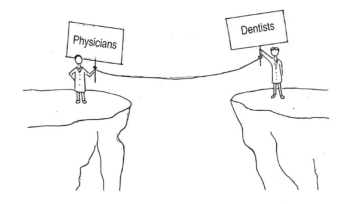

A Caring Cardiologist

While at dinner with a caring cardiologist, I asked, "If your patient had an infection in their leg or foot, would you operate on him?"

He replied, "Absolutely not."

I then asked, "What if it was in their arm or hand? Would that be okay?"

He quickly responded, "No. Absolutely not."

I then asked, "What if the infection is in their mouth? They don't know it and you don't know it. Are you still going to do surgery?"

My only regret is that I don't have a picture of his face after I asked him that question. This was a good cardiologist who truly cared for his patients. I could see the wheels turning in his brain. The next thing he said was perfect.

"All of our patients need a dental exam."

That's it! That's all we're asking. If 90% of dental infections have no pain, then without a thorough examination by a skilled dentist, there is no way to know whether the patient is safe for surgery or other treatment protocols that would otherwise be dangerous if accompanied by oral infections. If the examination finds no infection, great. Proceed with the next steps. However, if you discover a dental infection, you may have discovered the source of the medical issues. If you never identify the source, you'll treat the symptoms for the rest of your life. Knowing the source is key if your goal is to *cure* the disease. Remember the stories of Alice, Debbie, and Melissa from the last chapter? Once they restored oral health, no further treatments were needed.

When I ask physicians how much medical school training they received on the mouth, the usual answer varies from one day to one hour. That's all! I've often made a silly proposition to physicians: "If you believe your mouth is not part of your body, then when you go to work on Monday, leave your mouth at home."

You can't do it. The mouth *is* a vital part of the whole body no matter what we believe.

Speaking of belief, this brings us to an important topic: the difference between belief and truth.

Beliefs vs. Truths

I imagine you must be wondering, *Why are we talking about beliefs? I thought this book was about my teeth.* It is, but it is also about much more than teeth. This book is also about the beliefs that limit us.

When you ask people how often they should see their dentist, the stock answer is, "Twice a year." When you ask about brushing, almost everyone will say: "Brush twice a day." I wonder how many of us grew up with this belief, the origin of which came from a toothpaste commercial back in the 1940s. *There's nothing scientific about it.* The toothpaste company benefited because people went from brushing once to twice per day—doubling sales.

Ideas can stick even when they have no scientific basis and are just flat wrong. For how many centuries did people believe the world was flat? To the best of *their* knowledge, they were right. To the best of *our* knowledge, they were wrong. What you and I are discussing right now is more than a habit change. It is a paradigm shift. Few know about it; yet, it carries the power to transform the health of this generation. There is a real oral-systemic (mouth-body) connection, meaning that your mouth connects to all the systems of your body. Oral health affects overall health. What is happening in your teeth and gums touches your whole body, from how you look to how you feel.

Just because we believe something doesn't make it true. Over the centuries, countless beliefs have been proven incorrect. In the early 1900s, physicians believed that if a person traveled faster than 60mph, the wind would be sucked out from their lungs and they would suffocate. It may sound crazy today, but in a world where no one had traveled at that speed, people relied on the "experts." The belief prevailed until some brave soul tried it and survived.

You probably assume that washing your hands before performing surgery is common sense. However, until the late 1800s, physicians did not wash their hands between patients. They believed operating on people without first washing their hands was a perfectly safe practice. In fact, doctors routinely went from performing autopsies to delivering babies without washing their hands. This was not only a habit but a standard protocol.

In the 1840s, a Hungarian doctor named Ignaz Semmelweis was persecuted and even forced out of the medical society because he sincerely believed that this standard protocol was sincerely wrong.

Semmelweis watched as doctors moseyed along from opening up dead bodies to delivering babies from the womb—with unwashed hands. He observed that when midwives delivered babies their mortality rate was 36 babies per 1000 births. When doctors delivered babies, their mortality rate was 98 babies per 1000, three times the death rate of midwives.

The cause, Dr. Semmelweis determined, was "cadaveric matter," a fancy way of saying "stuff from dead bodies."

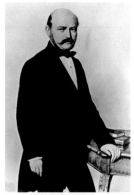

Dr. Ignaz Semmelweis

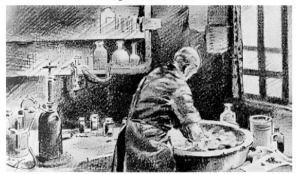

Dr. Ignaz Semmelweis

During the time of Doctor Ignaz Semmelweis, no one knew about bacteria. Doctors refused to believe that washing their hands was necessary. It took another 25 years before the medical communities reformed their belief to match the truth. How many babies died because of a false belief?

Beliefs can be strong and wrong all at the same time.

Today, a physician wouldn't think of delivering a baby or performing surgery without thoroughly washing their hands and wearing gloves. Truth wins over belief.

Are you old enough to remember when smoking tobacco was considered cool and sophisticated? Just because people believed cigarettes were safe didn't make them safe. The Marlboro Man, Joe Camel, Winston's, and many others were practically cultural icons. Commercials glamorized cigarettes. In 1964, the U.S. Surgeon General announced cigarettes were unhealthy; yet, even as warnings were heard it took one, maybe two generations for cigarette smoking to lose its luster to the general population. The people's beliefs led many to early graves and left many families devastated. Doctors even endorsed cigarettes for stress relief and recommended cigarettes during pregnancy. Today, we know that cigarettes are unhealthy, but physicians back then *believed* they supported health. Truth trumps belief.

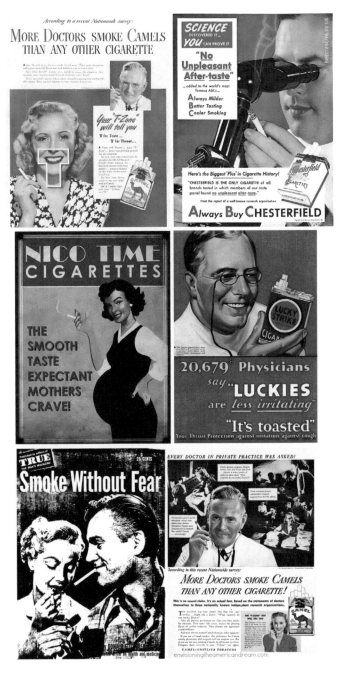

Many people believe that it is enough to see your dentist twice a year. As far as most of us know, that plan has proved sufficient. We haven't had any pain and can still comfortably chew food so we believe our mouth is healthy, but it is still a belief that may or may not be true.

It's probably not true.

According to the Centers for Disease Control, if you're over 30 there's a 47% chance you have symptom-free gum infections in your mouth right now. If you're over 65, the numbers jump to 70% have active gum disease, dumping harmful bacteria into the bloodstream.

After forty-plus years of dental practice, I believe those numbers are actually low. Most unchecked and untreated mouths have at least some form of dental disease, 90% of which, as I've stated, have no pain. Just because you don't hurt doesn't mean everything is healthy.

I've heard it said that people don't like to change their minds.

People will, however, make a new decision based on additional information.

In order for us to progress and evolve as a people, we must question our current beliefs. I hope reading this book gives you more than enough information to replace any harmful, limiting beliefs as you view your oral health from a whole new perspective.

People don't like to change their minds.
People will, however, make
New Decisions based on
Additional Information
This book is full of *additional information*
for you and your family.

Truth Trumps Tradition

You may have heard the story of the newlywed husband whose wife cooked a pot roast. Before she put the roast in the oven, she cut off an end and threw it away. Shocked, the young husband asked, "Why did you do that?"

She replied, "That's how my mother taught me to cook a roast."

Unsatisfied, the new husband went to his new mother-in-law and said, "I love your daughter so much, but when she cooks a roast, she cuts the end off and throws it away before putting it into the oven. She said she learned that from you. Is that right?"

His new mother-in-law replied, "Absolutely. That's the way my mother taught me to cook a roast."

Still unsatisfied with the answer, the new husband went to the grandmother and asked, "My beautiful new wife, your granddaughter, cooked a roast for us. Before she put the roast into the oven, she cut off an end and threw it away. She said she learned it from her mother, your daughter, who said she learned it from you. Is that true?"

"Mhmm," she replied.

"Why did you do that?" he asked.

The grandmother thought for a minute. Then she replied, "Our oven was really small, so I had to cut the end off to make it fit."

How many things do we believe today because that's the way we've always done it? Having a closed mind will get us into trouble. Tradition and old habits can severely limit our growth and even turn out to be deadly. Truth trumps tradition.

Oral Health and Surgery

If you have dental infections, your immune system is already working overtime trying to contain the problem and keep you healthy. Before undergoing surgery, it makes sense to have a healthy mouth. Otherwise, adding an invasive surgical procedure to an oral infection can overwhelm your immune system. When healthy immunity is compromised, healing becomes a painfully slow process and can lead to other vulnerabilities that make you sicker. It's not rocket science.

So, the final answer is: yes, your mouth is a crucial part of your body. As we've said, it isn't your physician's fault that your mouth isn't included in examinations, but that's why the information in this book is so vital to everyone—physicians included!

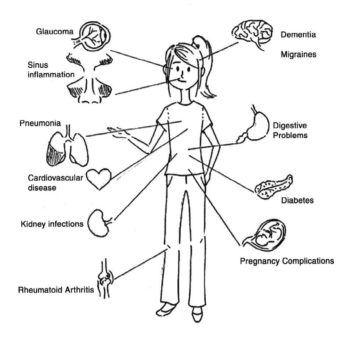

Let's review what we've learned so far:

1. The mouth is the front door to the body. Most bacteria enter the body through the front door. These bacteria cause or affect many medical problems: cardiovascular disease, heart attacks, strokes, E.D., diabetic and pregnancy complications, pneumonia, Alzheimer's disease, and rheumatoid arthritis. Lack of pain does not mean the mouth is healthy.

2. Most physicians were not trained to include the mouth as a part of a "complete" examination, but you can. You can bridge that deadly gap by choosing to have your mouth examined by a skilled dentist and then sharing the results of the oral exam with your physician. (We'll discuss how to share this information in Chapter 12).

Chapter 3

How to Fix the Deadly Gap
It's Simple, but Not Easy

Once doctors and patients recognize the oral-systemic connection, they will never consider an examination or treatment plan complete until the mouth has been checked. **Separating physicians from dentists and dentists from physicians has created a deadly gap that hurts both patients and physicians.**

None of this is new. Almost a century ago, physicians were connecting the dots between the mouth and our health.

In the 1934 edition of the Journal of the American Dental Association (JADA), in the article titled *Oral Infection in Relation to System Disease: Recent Studies (the viewpoint of an internist)*, a physician named Wilbur E. Post, MD, wrote:

"I cannot help thinking that our success in the treatment of all chronic diseases would be very much promoted, by directing our inquiries into the state of the teeth of sick people, and by advising their extraction in every case in which they are decayed. It is not necessary that they be attended by pain in order to produce disease."

This was a physician talking to the American Dental Association about the importance of dental health for general health. He even noted that you needn't suffer a toothache for a tooth to be diseased and affect your health. As I've repeated often, most dental infections have absolutely no pain.

In the year 2000, The Executive Summary of *Oral Health in America: A Report of the Surgeon* by David Satcher MD, PhD, Surgeon General, and the Secretary of Health and Human Services, Donna E. Shalala, stated:

"The terms oral health and general health should not be interpreted as separate entities. Oral health is integral to general health; this report provides important reminders that oral health means more than healthy teeth and that you cannot be healthy without oral health. Further, the report outlines existing safe and effective disease prevention measures that everyone can adopt to improve oral health and prevent disease."

Medical school doesn't teach physicians to refer dentists. Dentists seldom refer to physicians. Yet, both are working on the same body. Shouldn't we work together? It's been decades since the Surgeon General's report; nevertheless, there remains a deadly gap between physicians and dentists. Thankfully, by taking simple steps in this book and speaking with your healthcare professionals, you can eliminate that deadly gap for yourself and your family.

A Physician's Fresh Perspective

One of my patients was a physician. He was coming for an appointment not because of pain or knowledge of any infection, but because his teeth were getting loose. By the time he got to me, one tooth had literally fallen out. His appointment quickly morphed from an examination to a cosmetic emergency—he didn't want patients to see him with a missing front tooth. He was also diabetic. By the time we had his periodontal disease under control, he'd lost six teeth.

The oral infection had been contaminating his bloodstream for years. As a direct result of treating his gum disease, this doctor now reports having more energy and feeling better than he has in years. With his mouth in better health and no longer poisoning his bloodstream, he has found his diabetes is much more controllable. He learned firsthand the power of the oral-systemic connection, and how dramatically a healthy mouth can impact a patient's overall quality of life.

Just Ask Your Dog

Are there *any* doctors who include the mouth when performing an examination? Yes, and thank goodness! There is one group of doctors who have connected the dots between the mouth and the rest of the body for a long time—animal doctors: veterinarians.

Since dogs can't talk, vets must actively look for indications of health or disease. When you bring your dog to the veterinarian, one of the first things they look at is your dog's mouth. They know bad teeth cause dogs heart, kidney, and liver issues. If there's gum disease or tartar (calculus) buildup on the teeth, they recommend a dental cleaning to minimize the risk of other health challenges such as heart issues or kidney failure.

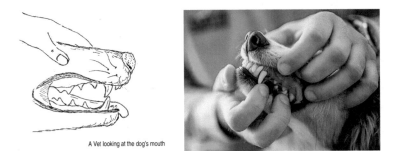

A Vet looking at the dog's mouth

To most, pets are like family members. Even though it takes $400-$600 for sedation and a dental cleaning, many people are willing to pay it because they don't want their best friend to be sick and in pain in the future.

Humans and dogs are both mammals. People have the same dental risks as dogs. Both have teeth, gums, hearts, lungs, kidneys, livers, and a blood supply that goes throughout the entire body. I asked my vet whether she ever reminded pet owners that dental infections pose the same risk in *their* mouths as in their pet's. She had never thought about it, but now she's joined us in spreading the oral-systemic message—to her *two-legged* clients.

You don't need a Hollywood smile to have a healthy mouth,

but you need a healthy mouth to have a healthy heart.

Many people believe you have to have a great smile to have a healthy mouth—not true. You don't even need to have teeth to have a healthy mouth! The teeth may be missing, stained, or crooked and yet be a healthy mouth. A person with no teeth and complete dentures could have a healthy mouth while another with a beautiful smile may have severe periodontal disease. Looks are deceiving. You can't judge the health of the mouth by the smile.

Common sense is so uncommon. Understanding the oral-systemic connection is not rocket science. It's common sense. The problem has been the deadly gap between physicians and dentists. It's time to close that gap so we can treat the whole person.

How Do We Close the Gap?

Trying to get physicians and dentists to work together has been like herding cats. I attempted to join the staff at our local hospital. My intent was to help identify oral infections so patients could rule out oral bacteria as a possible source of their medical issues.

The hospital staff replied, "We don't want you diagnosing things we can't treat."

I explained that I diagnose things I can't treat every week, so I refer my patients to someone who *can* treat them.

Their reply was, "We don't want to be in the referral business."

I was floored.

From there, I went to many physicians' offices encouraging them to include the mouth when evaluating a patient's health. I was then told that doctors barely had time to ask the required examination questions, much less the additional ones I was suggesting.

Dentists were not trained to share clinical findings with their patient's physician. Physicians were not trained to request a dental health report from their patient's dentist. The question for you and me isn't who is at fault, but rather where do we go from here? Seeing as physicians say they don't have the time or resources to cover this vital aspect of your health and quality of life, and some hospitals prefer not to, perhaps it is best for you and me to share this information with the world ourselves—one family at a time.

It Starts With You

When one person has a heart attack or stroke it doesn't affect just one person. It affects the entire family. It affects businesses and coworkers, friends and neighbors. Everybody's life is turned upside down when someone close to them falls severely ill. We've already covered that you can't rely on physicians or dentists to bridge this deadly gap for you.

Thankfully, taking action on what I've just told you empowers you to help avoid the medical, emotional, and financial tragedies followed by medical emergencies caused by painless dental infections. Simply opening the dialogue with your physician and dentist empowers you and your family. Families who take action can save themselves thousands of dollars in dental expenses and avoid easily preventable sicknesses that too often lead to medical issues or possibly even early death.

Ask Your Doctor(s)

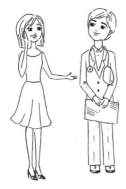

Don't wait for your physician(s) to ask about your dental health. During your next visit, ask your physician, "Does the health of my mouth have anything to do with the health of the rest of my body?" Be quiet and listen to their answer. You already know the answer. Absolutely it does! You want to find out what your doctor believes. Ask your dentist the same question.

If their answer is something like, "Yes, there's a big connection between dental health and medical health," you have a good doctor. Be thankful! Listen to their recommendations.

If their answer is more like, "Maybe, but I'm not sure," ask them to conduct a keyword search of "oral-systemic connections" or similar on the internet. Maybe find a study or great article and print or show it from your mobile device. There are hundreds of studies readily available. If your physician is open to gaining this new information, it's easy to get.

If their answer is, "No, there's no connection between the mouth and the rest of the body," you can decide if you want to keep that doctor or find another. It's *your* health we're interested in, and you need doctors, both physicians and dentists, who can see the bigger picture.

When doctors include the 5 Factors in Our Health mentioned in the Introduction (diet, exercise, a healthy mouth, a good night's sleep, and attitude) many more treatment options become available.

Cardiovascular disease, for instance, is reversible. With simple lifestyle changes, plaque in your arteries can be reduced. Diet, exercise, a healthy mouth, and a good night's sleep are essential for a healthy heart. Check the references in the appendix at the end of this book. You and your physician can also visit **www.TheDentalMedicalConvergence.org/doctors** for links to many research studies and articles establishing the connection between dental bacteria and systemic medical issues.

It's Family First!

Don't wait for your physician to ask you about your dental health. It is a huge factor in your overall health. Take the first steps. You can close the front door to unhealthy bacteria in your loved one's bloodstream. You can take control of your family's dental health, save thousands of dollars, and be healthier. Win, Win, Win!

Let's review what we've learned so far:

1. The mouth is the front door to the body. Most bacteria enter the body through the front door. These bacteria cause or affect many medical problems: cardiovascular disease, heart attacks, strokes, E.D., diabetic and pregnancy complications, pneumonia, Alzheimer's disease, and rheumatoid arthritis. Lack of pain does not mean the mouth is healthy.

2. Most physicians were not trained to include the mouth as a part of a "complete" examination, but you can. You can bridge that deadly gap by choosing to have your mouth examined by a skilled dentist and then sharing the results of the oral exam with your physician. (We'll discuss how to share this information in Chapter 12).

3. Ask your doctor(s) "Does the health of my mouth have anything to do with the health of the rest of my body?" You already know the answer. You want to see what your doctor believes.

Chapter 4

What's Your "WHY"?

If you don't know your "Why" you're risking failure

Goal #1 in oral care is to be fully clear of infections in your mouth. After that, different folks may have different goals—cosmetic or otherwise; but while goals are important, they are not the same as your *why*. Of all the questions we've asked thus far, "why" is by far the most important.

Why would you *want* to spend time every day thoroughly cleaning your teeth?

Connect to your *why*, and you'll have all the motivation you need to add oral care to your daily routine. If you're doing it to please someone else, you will eventually fail. You can't do it for them. You must do it for yourself. This is a very personal decision.

Heart Attack or Stroke Prevention

Maybe you want to avoid the trauma of a heart attack or stroke. Should you suffer such an event, your recovery could take weeks, months, or years, and even lead to permanent damage. The lives of those close to you will be suddenly consumed with caretaking.

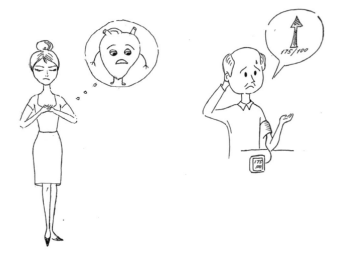

Perhaps the thought of debilitating medical expenses for doctor's visits, surgical procedures, and prescription drugs following a heart attack or stroke is enough to send you brushing.

According to cardiology researchers, 50% of strokes and heart attacks are triggered by dental infections. Please don't put your family members through caring for you for a completely avoidable situation. **It's not selfish to take care of your health.** In fact, one could argue that it *is* selfish to *not* take care of your own health. It's not a waste of time or resources to take preventive measures. It's smart and almost dirt cheap, especially compared to the potential care that would occur after serious dental infections and other problems. You can even start today with the free stuff at home (see Chapter 8 on homecare).

You don't need a Hollywood smile to have a healthy mouth, but you do need a healthy mouth to have a healthy heart.

Caring for Others

In my 40-plus years of dental practice, I found that caregivers—people taking care of others—had the hardest time caring for themselves. They were often so busy *giving* care that they didn't take the time to receive care. While the intention is certainly honorable, it isn't wise.

From the single mom to the son or daughter caring for their aged parent, I saw many a caregiver neglecting his/herself as they tended to their family. It may seem right at first, but remember: *when the workhorse goes down, everything stops.* Neglecting yourself eventually backfires. Realize now, before it's too late, that caring for yourself is not selfish. It's smart. It's what's best for your family, your job or career, and everyone your life touches. As you remain in good health, you remain good and able to continue as a caregiver, employee, CEO, or whatever keeps you galloping in life. That's not to mention all the money you'll save as you and your family maintain a healthy mouth, eliminating a common source of sickness and even early death.

For the caregiver, your "why" may be to continue caring for others. It could be taking steps to ensure you never become burdensome or staying healthy and strong to keep being the *rock* of the family that everyone counts on. The bottom line is that it is not selfish to care for your teeth and have a healthy mouth. It's smart!

Bad Breath

As a long-term mouth examiner, I promise you that clean mouths smell much better than dirty mouths. Maybe it's as simple as wanting fresh breath. We've all met people with bad breath. It can make your head spin. No one wants to be near you when your breath stinks. I've seen teeth with the tartar built up so thick you could hardly see the teeth anymore. You can imagine how all that buildup might make your mouth smell … and taste?

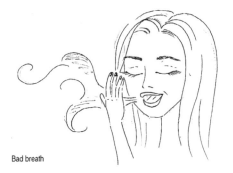

Bad breath

Gum disease has no pain. Most people have no idea when they have it, and 90% of bad breath comes from gum disease.

Have you ever met a cigarette smoker who was unable to smell cigarette smoke? They're called "nose blind." People can also be nose blind to *halitosis*, which is a fancy term for bad breath. People can be nose blind to cigarettes, body odor, bad breath, or any other bad smells they are exposed to on a long-term basis. Even some workplaces smell bad to others, but not to the people who work there. We adapt!

Gum disease bacteria cause cardiovascular disease, heart attacks, and strokes; worsen diabetes and rheumatoid arthritis; create complications during pregnancy; and are found in the brains of Alzheimer's patients.

If you notice someone with halitosis, it's okay to tell them in a caring way. If you speak with the right caring spirit and inform them of the connection between bad breath, gum disease, and other serious health complications, **you could save their life**. You don't have to engage in a heated debate. It's not your job to force them to take action. In Chapter 10, we'll cover your options for achieving a completely healthy mouth, which I'm happy to report are as easy as 1-2-3. The person will have to take ownership and do the work, but you can at least share the information; and if someone approaches to let you know that your breath is concerning, don't be offended. Thank them and go get it checked out. It could save *your* life.

Clean Feels Good

Maybe your reason for sticking with your few-minutes-per-day oral care plan is that you love the *feel* of a clean mouth!

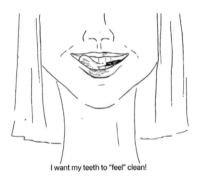

I want my teeth to "feel" clean!

Every time you eat, you get food stuck in your teeth. When you run your tongue around inside your mouth you can feel fuzzy stuff on your teeth. Ew! If that's your "why," then celebrate it. After you finish cleaning your teeth, slide your tongue around your teeth and celebrate that good clean feelin'. Smooth teeth … happy tongue … healthy mouth … feels great.

Start Here

Is the goal of a healthier mouth and fewer medical issues worth 8-10 minutes, once per day?

You're a pretty complex character. Take some time to think about why living a long, healthy life is important to you. Your reasons may be as unique as you are. You don't have to have it all figured out just to get started. You may find your "why" continues to grow and change over time. That's fine. What matters is that you don't just keep it in your head or write it down only to put it away as memorabilia in a shoebox, literally or figuratively. We'll get into the nitty-gritty of your daily routine in the next chapter; but if you answered "yes" to my last question, your first step and a key to your success start right here.

In Your Face Reminder

Once you determine your "why," draw a picture, find a symbol, write a few words or anything that visually reminds you of your "why," and put it in your face; that is, put it in a place where you will see it every day. I recommend attaching it to your bathroom mirror where you typically brush your teeth.

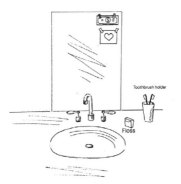

If health is your number one motivating factor, find a picture of a healthy heart or person. If you want to save money, tape a dollar bill to the mirror. Maybe a picture of your children or grandchildren will remind you why you are passionate about eliminating this one major hindrance to fulfilling your family-bliss dreams.

Whatever you decide, your "why" must be deeply important to you. Put it where you can't avoid seeing it so that it serves as a reminder to thoroughly clean your teeth once every day.

Let's review what we've learned so far:

1. The mouth is the front door to the body. Most bacteria enter the body through the front door. These bacteria cause or affect many medical problems: cardiovascular disease, heart attacks, strokes, E.D., diabetic and pregnancy complications, pneumonia, Alzheimer's disease, and rheumatoid arthritis. Lack of pain does not mean the mouth is healthy.

2. Most physicians were not trained to include the mouth as a part of a "complete" examination, but you can. You can bridge that deadly gap by choosing to have your mouth examined by a skilled dentist and then sharing the results of the oral exam with your physician. (We'll discuss how to share this information in Chapter 12).

3. Ask your doctor(s) "Does the health of my mouth have anything to do with the health of the rest of my body?" You already know the answer. You want to see what your doctor believes.

4. "Why" do I want a healthy mouth? Save money? Help prevent heart attacks, strokes, or other medical issues? Live longer? Know your *why*! Tape a motivating picture, photo, or money to your bathroom mirror.

Chapter 5

What Causes Cavities and Gum Disease?
It's Not Sugar!

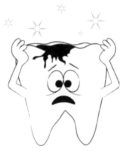

If cavities and gum disease dump bacteria into the bloodstream, what causes cavities and gum disease?

When asking my patients this question the #1 answer was always sugar. It's the wrong answer, but that's what most people believe.

Here's a pretty good analogy. To start a fire, we need three ingredients:

1. Fuel (wood, gas, etc)

2. Oxygen

3. An ignition source (match, spark)

If we remove any one of the ingredients, we cannot have a fire.

If you have no fuel, you have no fire. If you have no oxygen, you have no fire. If you have no ignition source, you have no fire.

If you have fuel and oxygen, but don't have an ignition source, it won't start on its own. If you have oxygen and an ignition source, but no fuel, you can't have a fire. If you have an ignition source and fuel, but no oxygen, you can't have a fire.

The same thing is true with cavities and gum disease—they require three ingredients:

1. A Tooth

2. Food

3. Bacteria

If you remove any one of these, you cannot have cavities or gum disease.

If you remove the tooth, you cannot have cavities or gum disease, but you won't have a tooth either.

If you remove the food, you cannot have cavities or gum disease, but you will die without food.

If you remove the bacteria, you cannot have cavities or gum disease.

Why is that?

When you and I eat food, the body makes byproducts. Namely, we poop and pee. When oral bacteria eat food, they also make byproducts, one of which is lactic acid.

When bacteria sticks to your teeth we call it plaque. These bacteria eat the foods we eat and then "poop" lactic acid. The acid is so strong it eats through (demineralizes) the teeth, eats through the enamel (small cavity), and into the next layer of the tooth, dentin (deeper cavity). There usually is no pain associated with this.

Cavities

If the plaque is not removed, the bacteria continue demineralizing and destroying the tooth structure. Once bacteria reach the middle (pulp) of the tooth, they gain access to the tooth's blood vessels and nerves, which provide a direct pathway into your bloodstream. As the bacteria invade the pulp of the tooth, they make their way down the root and into the bone surrounding the root. From there they continue destroying bone and invading the bloodstream.

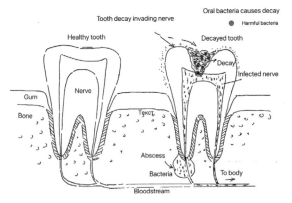

Gum Disease

As the bacteria work their way down the outside of the tooth and under the gum, your body wants to fight the invasion of harmful bacteria. The battlefield becomes the bone around your teeth. During the fight, the bone holding the tooth is slowly destroyed. There is no pain.

Eventually, enough bone is destroyed that the tooth gets loose. There is nothing wrong with the tooth, but the foundation that holds the tooth is destroyed.

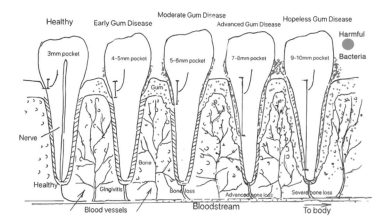

Like A Fence Post

A fence post with half of the fence post firmly underground will remain sturdy. However, if you took a garden hose and washed the dirt away from the bottom of the fence post, the post would be unstable, loosened, and eventually fall over. The fallen post remains in good condition, but its foundation was washed away and so the post fell out.

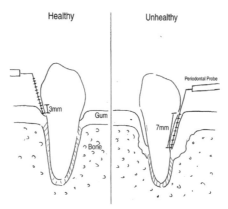

Healthy | Unhealthy

Periodontal Probe

3mm

Gum

7mm

Bone

It's the same with gum disease. The tooth may be perfectly fine, but if you lose the foundation, you lose the tooth. Losing the tooth isn't the worse part. The tooth can be replaced. Having harmful bacteria entering your bloodstream for the years that it takes to destroy the bone around your tooth is worse. *You can live without your teeth, but you can't live without your heart.* Certain oral bacteria have already been proven to cause cardiovascular disease.

How can we prevent cavities and gum disease?

1. Thoroughly remove the bacteria (plaque) that cause cavities and gum disease.

2. Limit sugar and carbohydrate intake.

3. Replenish good oral bacteria with oral probiotics.

Your body needs certain healthy bacteria in order for the body to do what it needs to do, including in the mouth. Many times the unhealthy oral bacteria overrun the healthy bacteria. So it's a good idea to replenish the good bacteria after we've thoroughly cleaned our teeth. Oral probiotics need to be dissolved in the mouth, directly on top of the teeth and gums, not swallowed. There are several oral probiotics available online. Check them out.

Now that you know what causes cavities and gum disease, and that the bacteria from cavities and gum disease cause or affect many medical conditions, you can begin connecting the dots between your oral health and the rest of your body. Once harmful oral bacteria hit your bloodstream, they're on the highway that leads to your heart, brain, pancreas, lungs— your whole body!

Chapter 6 goes into detail on how to thoroughly clean your teeth.

Let's review what we've learned so far:

1. The mouth is the front door to the body. Most bacteria enter the body through the front door. These bacteria cause or affect many medical problems: cardiovascular disease, heart attacks, strokes, E.D., diabetic and pregnancy complications, pneumonia, Alzheimer's disease, and rheumatoid arthritis. Lack of pain does not mean the mouth is healthy.

2. Most physicians were not trained to include the mouth as a part of a "complete" examination, but you can. You can bridge that deadly gap by choosing to have your mouth examined by a skilled dentist and then sharing the results of the oral exam with your physician. (We'll discuss how to share this information in Chapter 12).

3. Ask your doctor(s) "Does the health of my mouth have anything to do with the health of the rest of my body?" You already know the answer. You want to see what your doctor believes.

4. "Why" do I want a healthy mouth? Save money? Help prevent heart attacks, strokes, or other medical issues? Live longer? Know your *why*! Tape a motivating picture, photo, or money to your bathroom mirror.

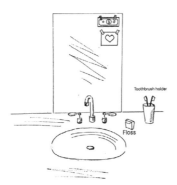

5. It isn't sugar that causes cavities and gum disease. It's bacteria eating the sugar dumping acid on the teeth and gums. Decreasing sugar, thoroughly removing dental plaque (bacteria), and adding an oral probiotic are the keys.

How to Thoroughly Clean Your Teeth
New Tricks

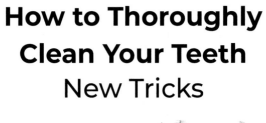

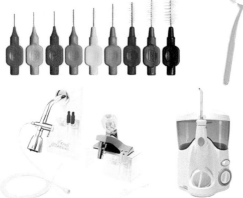

Taking care of your teeth at home is *free*. It takes a fairly small effort to properly clean your own teeth—you just need to know *how*. This chapter will answer that question.

It starts with building the habit.

We all have habits or routines we follow. If you're in the habit of placing your car keys inside a desk drawer next to your front entrance, it's likely you'll always find them there. If you're in the habit of drinking a cup of coffee first thing in the morning, it's unlikely you'll ever forget to make it. If you're in the habit of showing gratitude and appreciation to people, you'll end up with more friends. If you clean your mouth thoroughly every day, before too long you'll achieve a healthy "front door" to your body and avoid preventable sicknesses as a result.

Habits put results on autopilot.

Sometimes our habits bring about the results we want, and sometimes habits (or the lack thereof) bring results we don't want. Habits produced your current state, and developing these new habits will eventually produce a new state of health and well-being.

If the results you want on autopilot are

• a clean, healthy mouth that protects your body from preventable sickness and disease, and/or

• getting rid of bad breath, and/or

• saving thousands of dollars in medical expenses, and/or

• saving your loved ones from preventable sickness and injury

then the habit you want is a practice of cleaning your mouth for 8-10 minutes *one time* every day.

(And even if you don't have any teeth, keep reading; there is information here for you, too.)

One Hour to Paint the House?

The average person spends 30 seconds or less brushing their teeth. That's like saying, "I have an hour; I think I'll paint the whole house." You may throw some paint on the walls, but you're not going to do a very good job rushing.

Properly cleaning your teeth takes between 8-10 minutes *one* time a day. Even brushing 2-3 times per day is not necessarily effective. Once daily, done *right*, has proven far more effective than 2-3 times done wrong. Move too quickly, and you'll miss hunks of plaque and food debris.

Don't panic. You don't have to start at 8-10 minutes. You may start with 30 seconds and work your way up slowly. The key is to start somewhere and trust the process.

Tiny Habits, Huge Results

The easiest way to start a new habit is to build on an existing one. Start small. Incorporate your tiny change into your regular routine.

If you already brush your teeth quickly with a standard toothbrush, try brushing for 30 seconds longer.

If you already brush for a couple of minutes, start using an electric toothbrush, which is more efficient for removing plaque.

If you already use an electric toothbrush but you haven't been thorough with the backs of your teeth, add another 10-30 seconds to focus on brushing behind your teeth.

Where you begin is up to you. You want to start with something that you are 99.99% likely to actually *do*. If the task is too hard or too big, you'll know it quickly because, despite your best intentions and plans, you won't do it consistently.

The right tiny habit is the one you *will* do.

Once you do your tiny new habit consistently for a week or two, celebrate! Notice that feeling of satisfaction. It may have been a small habit, but it represents a HUGE win for you. With this new tiny habit established, both the habit and its results will be on autopilot. What's more, you'll have experienced successfully adding new tiny habits, and you'll know exactly how to do it again when you're ready to add the next one and stack your results.

Here are some ideas for tiny habits you might add to your routine, one habit at a time:

• Use an electric toothbrush.

• Extend your brushing time by increments of 30 seconds.

• Floss one tooth perfectly. Then move on to two teeth. Keep going.

Yes, you can start with just one tooth. We said to start small—and you can't get smaller than just one tooth! Decide which tooth you want to be completely clean. In the beginning, take whatever time you want. You'll increase that time when you're ready.

After you've completed your new routine and tiny habit, look in the mirror and give yourself a high five. When you look in the mirror and high-five yourself, it's almost as if you now have a partner to help you make the changes you want. (This is an idea from Mel Robbins. Check her out.) Do this every day and you'll be amazed at how it boosts your mood.

Morning, Noon, or Night: Just Do It Every Day!

You probably already brush your teeth at least once a day if you're reading this book. That's a good start. The easiest time to add cleaning between your teeth is just after you brush. You're already there, standing at the sink looking in the mirror, with all the supplies needed.

1. Look on the bathroom mirror where you posted your "why." It's a reminder and motivator!

2. Pull out your toothbrush, floss, interdental brush, Directed Water Irrigator (water floss), or whatever you use, and thoroughly clean just one tooth, being careful not to damage the tooth or gum.

Whatever your starting point, your goal is to eventually invest 8-10 minutes cleaning your mouth *one* time every day. You might prefer to clean your teeth in the morning. You might prefer before bed. Some will prefer to do both. You decide when you want to thoroughly clean your teeth.

It takes 24-36 hours for bacteria to accumulate to a sufficient level to damage your teeth or gums.

That's only one day! Thoroughly cleaning your teeth one time a day is much better than doing a poor job 2-3 times a day. You decide for yourself. Morning, evening, or both. Your choice!

Once you're used to thoroughly cleaning one tooth, you'll be ready to add more. Your level of satisfaction and protection from disease is directly proportional to the percentage of teeth you thoroughly clean. It may take a week or two for the first tiny habit to take root. That's okay. Once it's on autopilot, the habit ceases to be a chore. On your way to establishing the new habit, check and double-check your "why." Remind yourself this will save you pain and sickness, help you avoid medical issues, and keep a lot of money *in* your pocket. **Dental care is not expensive. Dental neglect is very expensive!** If you're traveling, you can still keep up with your tiny habit. Bacteria don't live in your home, but in your mouth; so, when you travel, you also have to clean your teeth.

It's not up to the insurance company, the government, your spouse, or your parents to clean your teeth. It's up to you. It's your body, hair, skin, and mouth. It's a very important part of you that needs attention every day. With it, you eat, talk, drink, and even kiss. It deserves some daily maintenance if you want it to last and serve as an effective barrier to infection in your body. Take pride and ownership of your mouth. Make and keep it healthy!

Home Inspection?

No, I'm not talking about having your home inspected but inspecting your own teeth *from* home. If you want to be sure you've removed all the bacteria from your teeth, you'll need to inspect your teeth after cleaning. The challenge is that plaque is the same color as your teeth. They may look clean, yet be covered in a plaque biofilm.

In order to see the plaque remaining on your teeth, use disclosing solution. You can buy it at most drug or grocery stores or online. It comes either as a rinse or a pill that you chew and spit out. Some disclosing solutions can mark plaque on your teeth pink, red, blue, or purple, depending on how old the plaque is. Pink is recent. Purple is old.

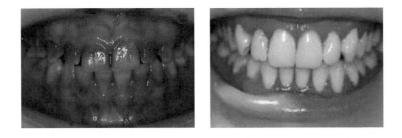

Clean your teeth as thoroughly as you can. Electric toothbrushes work best, but you can still do a good job with a manual toothbrush. It just takes longer.

How to Floss Properly

After you brush for at least two minutes, it's time to clean between your teeth. Little brushes are made that fit between your teeth called proxy brushes. Floss also works great—if you take your time and do it right. However, most people don't floss; they "pop." Popping is when you pop the floss between your teeth, wiggle it around a little, pop it out, and then pop between the next pair of teeth.

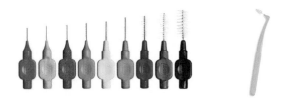

Instead of the "pop" method, which doesn't work well, flossing is when you pop the floss between two teeth, wrap the floss 180 degrees around one of those teeth, hug that tooth with the floss, slide the floss up and down several times, wrap it 180 degrees around the other tooth in the space, hug that tooth with the floss, slide the floss up and down several times, then pop it out and move on to the next space. Most people don't take the time to thoroughly floss their teeth like this. Most people are "poppers." If properly flossing is not easy for you, try using Directed Water Irrigation (DWI).

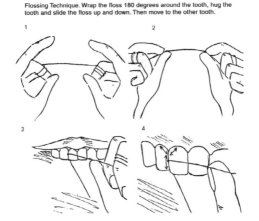

Flossing Technique. Wrap the floss 180 degrees around the tooth, hug the tooth and slide the floss up and down. Then move to the other tooth.

You can use DWI with a WaterPic, ShowerBreeze, or any device that shoots a stream of water. By shooting the water directly between the teeth and leaving the stream running for at least five seconds, you create a suction under the gums. This is a physics phenomenon called the *Venturi Effect*.

It's the suction that helps clean out to the bottom of the gum pocket, not the force of the water. The goal is to direct the water spray in the right direction to create a suction to clean out the gum pockets thoroughly.

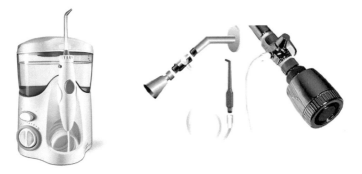

Thoroughly brushing, cleaning between your teeth (floss or DWI), and rinsing should take 8-10 minutes. If you have bridges or orthodontic braces, it will take longer, but the time you spend cleaning your teeth can save you cavities, gum disease, *time, money,* and *pain*. It's worth it, and it's only one time a day. Did I mention it's FREE?

The Problem with Mouthwash

What about mouth rinses? Will they help keep my mouth healthy?

Science has identified over 700 strains of bacteria in the mouth. Most of these are healthy for us and, in fact, we need them. There are only a handful that are harmful to us. Many bacteria are components of our immune system. To kill the good bacteria is to harm the immune system and make us more susceptible to illness.

When you use an antibacterial mouthwash, it doesn't differentiate between good and bad bacteria. It kills them all, which is not best for your health. Mouthwash is not the "silver bullet" for keeping your mouth healthy. It may make your mouth *feel* clean, but without removing the bacteria from your teeth, the mouthwash does little good and can actually do more harm by depleting your healthy bacteria.

Now that you've thoroughly removed the plaque from your teeth, replenish the good bacteria your mouth wants and needs by letting an oral probiotic dissolve in your mouth.

If you don't want to take the time to clean your teeth daily, don't complain about the cost of dental care. Remember, dental care isn't expensive. Dental *neglect* is very expensive. Start your new habit today and reap the rewards!

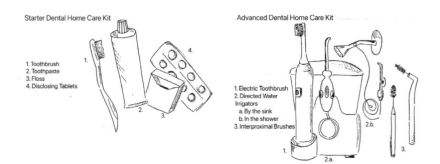

Starter Dental Home Care Kit

1. Toothbrush
2. Toothpaste
3. Floss
4. Disclosing Tablets

Advanced Dental Home Care Kit

1. Electric Toothbrush
2. Directed Water Irrigators
   a. By the sink
   b. In the shower
3. Interproximal Brushes

Let's review what we've learned so far:

1. The mouth is the front door to the body. Most bacteria enter the body through the front door. These bacteria cause or affect many medical problems: cardiovascular disease, heart attacks, strokes, E.D., diabetic and pregnancy complications, pneumonia, Alzheimer's disease, and rheumatoid arthritis. Lack of pain does not mean the mouth is healthy.

2. Most physicians were not trained to include the mouth as a part of a "complete" examination, but you can. You can bridge that deadly gap by choosing to have your mouth examined by a skilled dentist and then sharing the results of the oral exam with your physician. (We'll discuss how to share this information in Chapter 12).

3. Ask your doctor(s) "Does the health of my mouth have anything to do with the health of the rest of my body?" You already know the answer. You want to see what your doctor believes.

4. "Why" do I want a healthy mouth? Save money? Help prevent heart attacks, strokes, or other medical issues? Live longer? Know your *why*! Tape a motivating picture, photo, or money to your bathroom mirror.

5. It isn't sugar that causes cavities and gum disease. It's bacteria eating the sugar dumping acid on the teeth and gums. Decreasing sugar, thoroughly removing dental plaque (bacteria), and adding an oral probiotic are the keys.

6. How to clean your teeth involves removing the bacteria from the teeth without damaging the tooth or the gum. Tools: toothbrush, electric toothbrush, floss, interdental brushes, Directed Water Irrigation, Disclosing Tablets or Solution. Take 8-10 minutes one time a day.

Chapter 7

Kids
Is There Hope?

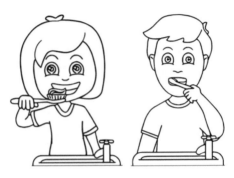

How do you get kids and teenagers to want to clean their teeth?

It's a struggle. Sometimes it can be unpleasant, a fight, and certainly a challenge to get your children of all ages to "brush your teeth." The more you push, the more they resist. Wouldn't it make your life much easier if your kids "wanted" to clean their teeth? We've heard the phrase, "You can lead a horse to water, but you can't make him drink." That may be true, but you can make him thirsty. Once he's thirsty, he'll want to drink.

The same is true with kids from two to ninety-two. How do you make kids of all ages *thirsty* so they want to clean their teeth? There is no single answer. It all depends on what triggers their *wants*. Figure out your child's "why" and you'll know just how to help them do all the right things for them to succeed at achieving it.

Much of that depends on their age, however, and will change as they grow.

Kids: Is There Hope?

What we want changes through life. Children want different things than adults. Adults want different things than children. The same thing is true of what we *don't want*. Children don't want certain things (certain foods, baths, an early bedtime) and adults don't want other things (debt, health issues, rejection).

So, how do you make children thirsty or, in other words, *want* to clean their teeth? No doubt, you know how to create incentives and define consequences, but you might also tell them this story. It's completely true, and it's in language children will understand.

Poop in My Mouth?

Everybody has tiny little animals in our mouths that like to stick to our teeth called "Sugar Bugs." These Sugar Bugs are really tiny, almost invisible, and very nasty. You want to get these bugs off your teeth because, if you don't, while you're asleep, they poop all over your teeth.

A Simple Guide to a Healthy Smile

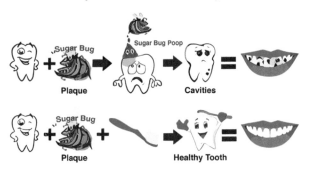

The Sugar Bug poop is so nasty, it eats holes into your teeth ... cavities. If you wake up in the morning and your mouth tastes really bad, it's probably Sugar Bug poop.

Kids may not understand bacteria, but they do understand POOP and don't want poop in their mouths.

Plus, it's all true! Bacteria (Sugar Bugs) stick to your teeth. We call this "plaque." When the bacteria (Sugar Bugs) eat foods that we have in our mouths (sugary food is worse), they produce byproducts (poop). One of the ingredients in the poop is lactic acid. Lactic acid demineralizes tooth enamel and causes cavities (holes) in the teeth. If we don't clean off the Sugar Bugs, the cavities (holes) get bigger and you will need fillings, root canals, or extractions. Sometimes, but not always, there will also be a toothache. Most kids don't want fillings or extractions. They don't want pain either.

You can take the unwanted—Sugar Bug poop, fillings, extractions, and pain—and turn them into wants. They *want* to get the Sugar Bugs off their teeth because they don't want poop in their mouth. They may not have yet experienced a toothache and so have no reference point, but if they have had one, they will want to avoid dental pain again.

Ages 0-6

The key to your child's lifelong dental health is to begin the habit of daily and thoroughly cleaning their teeth as soon as teeth erupt. Remove plaque or "poop" and those pesky Sugar Bugs without damaging the teeth or gums. The earlier and more consistently you begin thorough daily cleanings, the more easily it will be established as *their* daily routine. This is what you want. You want oral care to be a normal, expected part of the day so that, by the time your child is old enough to clean their own teeth, oral care is on autopilot. Nevertheless, until a child is about six years old, they don't have the skills to properly clean their own teeth. It's up to the parents or caregivers.

The good news is that it doesn't have to be complicated. You just do the same thing, preferably at the same time every day, and by the time the child is ready to try it on their own, they will be intimately acquainted with the process. At first, you'll need to supervise and check their work. It may also support their good habit if you perform your oral care routines together each and every day.

Checking Your Work

As we discussed earlier, Sugar Bugs in the plaque are the same color as your teeth. You can't see them with the naked eye, so how can you check to see whether the bugs were sufficiently removed? Enter the disclosing solution from the last chapter.

First, clean your teeth as thoroughly as you can. Then, for younger children, paint disclosing solution on their teeth using a cotton-tipped applicator (you'll need the liquid disclosing solution instead of the tablets for this). Then, rinse out their mouth with water. Wherever bacteria remains, you will see a stain on the teeth. The stain doesn't indicate that you didn't brush the tooth. It means the brushing didn't remove all the bacterial plaque.

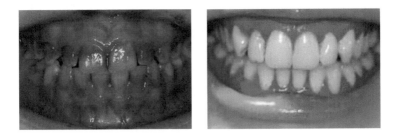

Wherever there is a stain, simply go back and clean it off the tooth again. This process teaches you what it takes to thoroughly clean your teeth.

Ages 7-12

From ages 7-12, many children go through the "ugly duckling" stage. Their teeth appear to be too big for their head. There are gaps where baby teeth have come out. Children of this age don't worry about their dental appearance as much because their peers are having the same experience. At this stage, just keep an eye on proper tooth alignment as adult teeth begin erupting. If there's enough space, the adult tooth comes in where it should—where the baby tooth was lost. If there's not enough space, the adult tooth may not erupt properly, producing crooked teeth. The sooner you can address the crooked teeth the better the final result.

Thoroughly cleaning these teeth once a day is critical. There are more hiding places for the plaque (bacteria) to gather during this "ugly duckling" stage.

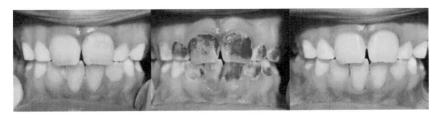

Make a game out of it. Once a week have a contest. The whole family, or whomever you can get to participate, has a competition. Everybody meets in the bathroom. Mom, Dad, brothers and sisters each clean their teeth as thoroughly as they can on their own. Then they chew a disclosing tablet and rinse out their mouths. Whoever has the least amount of stain on their teeth after using disclosing solution gets a prize. The prize can be a game, staying up later, or even cash. It's good for the kids to see that Mom or Dad have to spend time cleaning their own teeth as well. And if your kids are doing a great job cleaning their teeth, make it a good prize. That's money you won't have to spend at the dentist's!

Teens

A few fillings and some homecare instruction can turn a child's life completely around. Feeling good about your teeth and smile is important for the next phase: the teenage years. When children enter their teenage years, their *wants* and *don't wants* change. They grow more interested in how other people feel about them. They want other people to accept them. They don't want rejection. What can make teenagers reject other teenagers?

Bad teeth can create negative press in a teenager's life. Studies show that the first thing people notice about other people is their face. On their face, the first thing noticed are the teeth and the second are the eyes. You can show emotion with both the mouth and eyes. A nice smile makes a person more approachable. A bad smile makes a person less approachable. It may not be fair, but it's true. The same thing is true about BREATH!

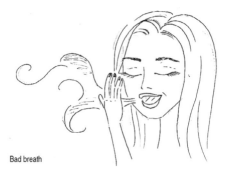

Bad breath

We've said that the number one reason for bad breath is gum disease, which has no pain, but it does have consequences. For teenagers, bad breath may be detrimental to their social life. People tend to avoid other people who have bad breath. Besides the breath, gum disease causes the bone to be destroyed around the teeth leading to eventual tooth loss if left untreated.

If teenagers want acceptance, a healthy smile will help greatly. That alone will be enough motivation for many teenagers to spend more time thoroughly cleaning their teeth on a daily basis.

People with a great smile are innately assumed to be more intelligent, trustworthy, clean, successful, educated, and honest. People with a bad smile are, unfortunately, judged as dirty, dishonest, uneducated, untrustworthy, diseased, or on drugs. The unconscious thought that comes up automatically in many people's minds is, "If they let their mouth get so bad, what about the rest of their body?"

Take advantage of what your teenagers *want*. Remember being a teenager? It's a difficult phase in life. Let them know how a healthy mouth and a good smile will boost their lives socially and otherwise.

A great smile opens many doors!

Let's review what we've learned so far:

1. The mouth is the front door to the body. Most bacteria enter the body through the front door. These bacteria cause or affect many medical problems: cardiovascular disease, heart attacks, strokes, E.D., diabetic and pregnancy complications, pneumonia, Alzheimer's disease, and rheumatoid arthritis. Lack of pain does not mean the mouth is healthy.

2. Most physicians were not trained to include the mouth as a part of a "complete" examination, but you can. You can bridge that deadly gap by choosing to have your mouth examined by a skilled dentist and then shar-

ing the results of the oral exam with your physician. (We'll discuss how to share this information in Chapter 12).

3. Ask your doctor(s) "Does the health of my mouth have anything to do with the health of the rest of my body?" You already know the answer. You want to see what your doctor believes.

4. "Why" do I want a healthy mouth? Save money? Help prevent heart attacks, strokes, or other medical issues? Live longer? Know your *why*! Tape a motivating picture, photo, or money to your bathroom mirror.

5. It isn't sugar that causes cavities and gum disease. It's bacteria eating the sugar dumping acid on the teeth and gums. Decreasing sugar, thoroughly removing dental plaque (bacteria), and adding an oral probiotic are the keys.

6. How to clean your teeth involves removing the bacteria from the teeth without damaging the tooth or the gum. Tools: toothbrush, electric toothbrush, floss, interdental brushes, Directed Water Irrigation, Disclosing Tablets or Solution. Take 8-10 minutes one time a day.

7. Find the age-appropriate motivating factors. Sugar Bugs, sex appeal, or health. What do they "Want" or "Don't Want"?

Chapter 8

How to Find a Good Dentist
Look Before You Leap

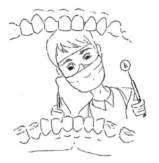

As we've discussed, your dental health is critical to your well-being. It stands to reason, then, that selecting a good dentist is critical to your overall health as well.

Within any profession, you will find that some are better than others. Not all dentists can offer you the same quality of care, attention, or results. Whether physicians, attorneys, electricians, plumbers, or dentists, there are always good and other-than-good ones you could hire. The quality of dentistry is up to the dentist, period. It's not up to the insurance company, dental assistants, or the dentist's employer if they are an employee. Your goal is to find someone who cares about your *health*, not just what's in your wallet.

A Few Shopping Tips

If you haven't yet selected a family dentist you trust, it's a good idea to do a little digging *before* you or someone you love begins treatment. Here are some steps. If you already have a good dentist, great! Be thankful.

First, a New Patient Examination costs $100-$350 or more. If you have dental insurance, it will only cover the *first* dental examination. The other examinations are paid out-of-pocket. Choose wisely. Start with a list of three or more potential dentists. Ask your local friends with healthy mouths what dentist they use. Look at online reviews. You're looking for the dentist that will be best for you.

Beware of "free" first visits. They might not be as thorough as you need to discover hidden, symptom-free dental infections.

Second, schedule your appointments.

Third, show up! Listen closely to the dentist's reasons for their treatment recommendations. Compare the different treatment plans at home. If you have additional questions, call the dental office for clarification.

Dentist examining mouth

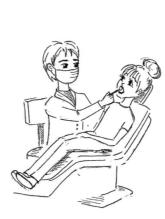

What to Expect

From any qualified dentist, you can expect a thorough examination including:

• Review of medical history, dental history, and current mediations

• X-rays

• Soft tissue examination, cheeks, lips, tongue, etc.

• Measure gum pockets

• Check the bite

- Discuss airway restrictions or related conditions such as Sleep Apnea (snoring)

- Discuss saliva testing in the case of cavities or infections

Following the examination, the dentist should be able to share their assessments about the health of your mouth, followed by recommendations for your treatment.

After your first visit with Dentist #1, do the same with Dentists #2 and #3. Second and third opinions have great value. Notice similarities and differences in their assessments and treatment recommendations—and ask questions. You can always call the office with your inquiries after you've gathered more information. You can also request copies of your X-rays to send to Dentist #2 and #3 to save both expense and exposure, although with digital X-rays there is very little exposure. Digital X-rays can be emailed and shared with other dentists.

It may take several auditions before you find the dentist you trust. The money you spend searching will be money well spent, especially when you consider the consequences of having the wrong dentist perform unnecessary procedures. Just like you can't "un-ring" a bell, often once an oral procedure is done, it can't be undone.

Do some research. Ask friends for referrals. Listen to your gut. Find the right dentist for YOU.

> Find a dentist you trust, then let them do their job.
> If you don't trust them, look for another dentist.

And if you already have a great dentist, that's super! Celebrate! Many people are still looking for a dentist they can trust.

Do It in Phases

Question: How do you eat an elephant?

Answer: One bite at a time!

If your trusted dentist prescribes a large treatment plan, don't be overwhelmed. You can break it into phases starting with treatments most vital to your health and working your way into more cosmetic concerns.

Phase I: Get Rid of Infections

Your number one goal at the beginning of your treatment is to get rid of tooth and gum infections. Unless there is trauma or some other emergency, ridding the mouth of infections is a cornerstone to a healthy mouth and healthier body. This may involve gum treatment, root canals, and/or extractions.

When you rid your mouth of otherwise painless dental infections that have been taxing your immune system, you will often experience more energy. The immune system gets to rest, replenish, and tend to other matters like keeping you resistant to infection, freeing up energy, and generally making you feel a whole lot better.

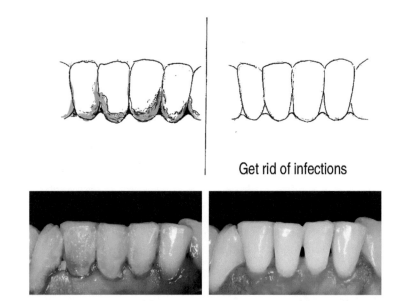

Get rid of infections

Phase II: Restore Teeth & Smile

The next phase may include restoring weak or broken teeth, replacing missing teeth, or simply improving your smile. These are all important but far secondary to removing infections that dump harmful bacteria into your bloodstream leading to systemic diseases, diseases that don't just affect one part or organ, but the whole body.

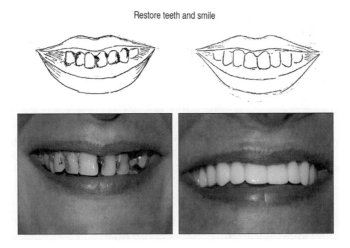

Restore teeth and smile

The Price is ... Right?

When people mistakenly believe all dentists are basically the same, their next mistake is often to choose based on the cheapest bidder. Years ago, my grandfather taught me a valuable lesson. I was buying a new belt because my old one was breaking apart. My grandfather showed me his. He asked, "How old do you think this belt is?"

It looked brand new.

He said, "It's over twenty years old."

He asked me how much I thought he paid for it. I had no idea. He said he paid $10 for that twenty-year-old belt in 1945 when $10 was a lot of money. It was now 1965 and the belt still looked brand new.

What he said next is with me to this day: **"The quality is remembered long after the price is forgotten."** Many times "cheap" ends up being "more expensive" in the long run.

This is business. Get a written estimate for your dental care.

I was often shocked as patients brought me estimates from another dental office. If the patient's goal was to have a healthy mouth, why was the treatment plan and cost estimate built for a Hollywood smile? Cases like that demonstrate why second and third opinions are invaluable.

Keep in mind the dentist's estimate is only an estimate. Some dentists quote on the higher side so as not to hit you with an unpleasant surprise later; but, there are also some who lowball the costs just to gain your patronage. Again, that is why you're doing your research.

Also, X-rays don't show everything and there could be a surprise once treatment begins. The possible additional fees should be discussed *before* any treatment is started. Personally, I always gave the estimate on the high side. If your car mechanic estimated $1,000 in repairs but only charges you $800 once the work was done, you'll leave a happy camper and will be likely to return. That was my approach. Not all dentists think like I do, though, so be aware that the estimate is just an estimate.

The most expensive is not necessarily the best. The cheapest price might not be the best deal either when you consider the repercussions of cheap work done with cheaper materials. Do your research. Read the reviews. Ask around. Price is not a reliable measure. You'll need to dig a little deeper, but I know without a doubt you can do it!

Once you've gathered information from your potential dentists, you can easily compare treatment plans and estimated costs.

Not on Your Insurance?

In the United States, you can legally see any dentist you want. Don't let your insurance company dictate to whom you entrust your life and well-being.

Just because they're on the insurance list doesn't mean they're right for you. Most insurance companies will pay for an out-of-network dentist. True, sometimes you'll pay more; other times, you might pay exactly the same or even less money than you would for the in-network dentist. It all depends on the recommended treatment. Do your research.

For instance, if your seven-year-old is like many her age, she may need a cleaning and a few fillings. On the other hand, she might not need any fillings. Not infrequently, a seven-year-old child will need ten or more fillings. These factors will impact the cost of care, which is why it will be worth your while to get opinions from several dentists.

If you have children, once you've found the dentist or dental office you trust, let them treat you and your whole family. If the children are young, they may need a pedodontist (pediatric dentist), but many general dentists also treat children, so it's good to ask.

I'm repeating myself, but please remember that 90% of dental infections have no pain. You need a dentist who will thoroughly examine your mouth to make sure you're disease free.

Support for Homecare

Remember that hiring a dentist is not a replacement for homecare, and homecare is not a replacement for hiring a dentist. You need both for optimal health. Whether your dentist is in-network or out-of-network; whether they are high priced or reasonably priced; in general, your dentist should do these three things well:

• Perform a proper dental examination

• Offer treatment options that you can break into phases if needed

• Explain and, if necessary, teach you proper homecare to prevent oral disease and maintain a healthy mouth

Ultimately, it's what you do at home that will make or break your dental health plan. As I've told my patients many times before:

"The more time you spend at home thoroughly cleaning your teeth, the less time you'll spend in a dental chair. The less time you spend at home thoroughly cleaning your teeth, the more time you spend in a dental chair, the more money it will cost you, and the more damage you do to your body."

My goal is to do less dental treatment and take less money from patients and to achieve that patients must do a few things for a few minutes daily to maintain oral health. A great dentist will equip and encourage you to do the necessary oral maintenance at home. They will make themselves available for periodic oral examinations and professional cleanings at the dental office or have some way of ensuring you get regular care according to their plan for you.

If the dentist recommends a three-month frequency for professional dental cleanings but they don't have available appointments, you may have to consider alternatives. Some patients alternate between a periodontist (a gum specialist) and their regular dentist. Some patients offer to be "on call" so they are quickly notified when a hygiene appointment becomes available.

However you deal with it, be proactive. Make it your goal to do the homecare and do it every day. Select a dentist you can trust, and then trust them to do their job. Your mouth is the front door to your body. Keep it clean and healthy.

Let's review what we've learned so far:

1. The mouth is the front door to the body. Most bacteria enter the body through the front door. These bacteria cause or affect many medical problems: cardiovascular disease, heart attacks, strokes, E.D., diabetic and pregnancy complications, pneumonia, Alzheimer's disease, and rheumatoid arthritis. Lack of pain does not mean the mouth is healthy.

2. Most physicians were not trained to include the mouth as a part of a "complete" examination, but you can. You can bridge that deadly gap by choosing to have your mouth examined by a skilled dentist and then sharing the results of the oral exam with your physician. (We'll discuss how to share this information in Chapter 12).

3. Ask your doctor(s) "Does the health of my mouth have anything to do with the health of the rest of my body?" You already know the answer. You want to see what your doctor believes.

4. "Why" do I want a healthy mouth? Save money? Help prevent heart attacks, strokes, or other medical issues? Live longer? Know your why! Tape a motivating picture, photo, or money to your bathroom mirror.

5. It isn't sugar that causes cavities and gum disease. It's bacteria eating the sugar dumping acid on the teeth and gums. Decreasing sugar, thoroughly removing dental plaque (bacteria), and adding an oral probiotic are the keys.

6. How to clean your teeth involves removing the bacteria from the teeth without damaging the tooth or the gum. Tools: toothbrush, electric toothbrush, floss, interdental brushes, Directed Water Irrigation, Disclosing Tablets or Solution. Take 8-10 minutes one time a day.

7. Find the age-appropriate motivating factors. Sugar Bugs, sex appeal, or health. What do they "Want" or "Don't Want"?

8. Finding the right dentist for you and your family may take some work. You may have to visit several dentists before you find the dentist you are comfortable with and trust. The money you spend on finding the right dentist is money well spent.

Chapter 9

My Dental Exam
What's Involved and Will It Hurt?

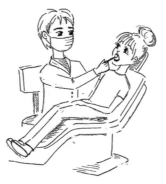

One of my patients had a brother-in-law who hadn't seen a dentist for years. One day, he decided to get his teeth checked. The dentist conducted an exam and then referred him to an oral surgeon. The oral surgeon conducted an exam, ran a few tests, and then informed the patient that he had about two months to live due to oral cancer. He died five days later.

Being in a dentist's chair should not be painful. As we've discussed, methods have improved greatly. On the other hand, never going because you're not sure what to expect or because you're nervous about discomfort can be deadly—literally. After all, a complete dental exam done at a much earlier stage might have saved that man's life.

These are the benefits of an excellent, potentially life-saving oral exam. I hope that knowing what to expect will prepare you and help alleviate any jitters as you discover that the procedures are better than they used to be, and constantly improving.

Ch-Ch-Ch-Changes!

My, how times have changed in dentistry. It used to be that a few X-rays and a look around your mouth were the extent of your dental exam. When I graduated dental school in 1979, we had panoramic X-rays that showed your jaw joint (TMJ), sinuses, and the complete mandible (lower jaw). We looked for cavities. Bitewing X-rays showed them between your teeth. As far as we knew at the time, if the sharp explorer stuck in your tooth, it was a cavity. If it didn't, it wasn't a cavity.

We checked your bite to make sure your teeth were lining up correctly. We used a periodontal probe to measure gum "pockets" around your teeth. The deeper the pocket, the weaker the support surrounding the tooth. Pockets had to be checked to ensure adequate support for a tooth before performing certain procedures such as placing a new cap (crown). We did all that back then but today, we have new techniques, equipment, and methods for a more complete examination.

Four Key Areas

Today, we start by reviewing your medical, dental, and medication history. We look for red flags including a history of cardiovascular concerns including stents, heart attack, high blood pressure, or strokes, as well as other concerns like diabetes, rheumatoid arthritis, or a pregnancy complication. There could be a dental component to each of these conditions, so we must examine your mouth carefully to either confirm or rule out a dental source for the disease.

Once we have an overview of your history, there are four key areas of oral health your dentist must examine:

1. Infections

2. Airway Restriction

3. Occlusion (Bite)

4. Oral Cancer

With today's improved diagnostic methods and tools for examination, dentists can obtain a detailed and comprehensive overview of your current oral and overall health.

Blood Pressure & Pulse

For years I didn't check blood pressure because of something often called "white coat syndrome," which is elevated blood pressure due to the anxiety people feel about being in a dentist's or doctor's office. Later, I learned that if your blood pressure is elevated just from being in a dental office, it's probably elevated during other stressful situations like driving on the highway or watching the news. In 2019, my suspicions were confirmed as researchers at Penn Medicine published a study in the Annals of Internal Medicine with significant findings "that patients with untreated white coat hypertension not only have a heightened risk of heart disease, but they are twice as likely to die from heart disease than people with normal blood pressure."

It's important to know if you have episodic high blood pressure; it's worth getting checked out—even at the dentist's office.

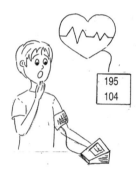

Blood pressure checking/ high blood pressure

X-Rays

Today's X-rays are safer. Hopefully, your dentist uses digital X-rays, which use a fraction of the radiation of the old film techniques. In addition to lower radiation, digital X-rays make it a snap for your dentist to email images to a specialist for a faster second opinion. We can enlarge or even colorize the images to clearly view details that were otherwise difficult to see, such as changes in tooth or bone density, or radiolucency. CBCT or 3D radiographs are now available that show much more than traditional two-dimensional radiographs. These are often used when placing implants or identifying tumors, tooth abscesses, or other lesions. They also allow you to check for airway restrictions for sleep apnea.

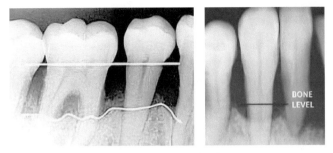

x-ray shows bone loss under the gums

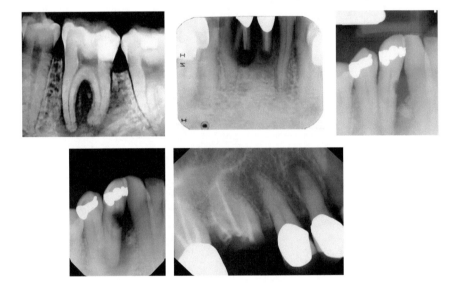

Photographs

Photographs are an excellent way to show a patient what is happening inside their mouth. Small intra-oral cameras photograph individual teeth, fillings, cracks, cavities, broken teeth, stains, recession, wear, puffy gums, or local infections.

Extra-oral cameras, which are outside your mouth, show different angles of your smile. Using external cameras allows us to see your complete dental arches. This shows teeth alignment—missing, tipped, or rotated teeth—and the roof and the floor of your mouth. A picture is worth a thousand words. Most patients have never seen their teeth this way. These pictures also make for excellent before-and-after records as we watch for changes in your mouth over time.

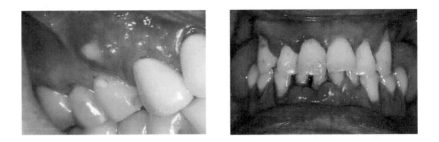

Gum Pockets

Periodontal probing is a term for measuring the depth of the sulcus, or gum pocket, between your tooth and gum. In a healthy mouth, these pockets are 1-3 millimeters deep. As the pocket deepens to 4mm, 5mm, 6mm, or more, the periodontal disease gets worse.

Remember the fence post metaphor I used previously? If you wash the dirt away from the bottom of the fence post, the post finds itself in shallow ground and eventually falls over. The fence post is fine. It falls out because the foundation was washed away.

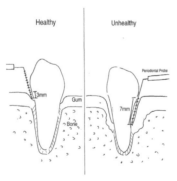

Stages of Gum Disease and Pocket Depth

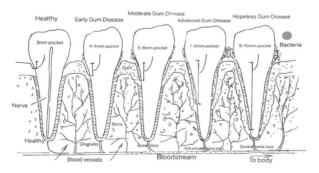

Gum disease works the same way. Although you don't have a garden hose in your mouth, you do have plaque—the bacteria that deposit acids and other toxins around your tooth. This ignites a great battle as your body comes under attack from bacteria and toxins. The bone around your tooth becomes the battlefield, destroying it in the process. As the bone is destroyed, the pocket gets deeper and deeper until, just like the fence post, your tooth loosens and falls out.

Worse than losing your teeth is the infection that is absorbed into your bloodstream and spreads throughout your whole body.

I'm still amazed when patients tell me they have never had their gum pocket depths checked by a dentist. Periodontal probing has been taught for many decades. I was taught in 1979 to check the pocket depths on every patient. It is a vital component of your complete dental exam. In fact, without it, you technically have not had a *complete* dental exam at all.

Cavities, Decay, and DIAGNOdent

As mentioned earlier, dentists were taught that if the sharp explorer didn't stick in the tooth, it wasn't a cavity. WRONG! Many times, the explorer wouldn't stick despite decay under the enamel.

Today we have DIAGNOdent, a laser cavity detector, that can look *through* the enamel for decay. It can also detect the difference between stain and decay, which is important because a dark spot on a tooth doesn't automatically mean it's a cavity. The DIAGNOdent helps prevent unnecessary fillings as well as discover previously undetectable decay.

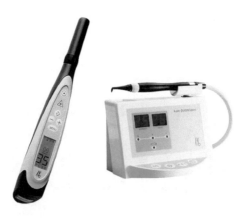

Saliva Testing

What bacteria are in *your* mouth? We don't all have the same bacteria in our mouths. Saliva testing identifies your unique mouth bacteria so that if you have gum disease, we know which antibiotics to add to your oral rinses. It's a big help toward getting your mouth healthy, and quicker, too. Saliva testing can also check for HPV viruses and soon will be able to identify certain cancers, such as lung cancer.

The rest of your complete dental exam is looking for airway restrictions, evaluating your bite, and checking for signs of oral cancer.

Oral Cancer

Oral cancer is on the rise. In the United States, one person dies from oral cancer *every hour*. One of our biggest challenges is that this cancer comes with no symptoms. As with high blood pressure, diabetes, and glaucoma, the disease doesn't hurt until it's too late.

Part of your complete dental exam is an oral cancer exam. We look at your throat, the hard and soft palate, cheeks, tongue, floor of the mouth, and lips.

There are special lights and rinses available to show oral cancer before it's visible in normal light. Velscope is one such light. It can show where cells are multiplying faster than the cells around them, even when they look normal to the naked eye. Since we don't yet know how to prevent oral cancer, early detection is the next best thing.

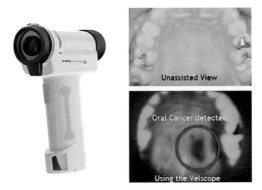

Unassisted View

Oral Cancer detected

Using the Velscope

Sleep Apnea

Over twenty million Americans have some type of Sleep Disordered Breathing, or sleep apnea, and only one in ten has any idea. Sleep apnea robs the body of the needed rest and repair that takes place when we're in deep sleep. 90% of people are unaware they suffer from sleep apnea. If you are likely to nod off or fall asleep when you're reading a book, watching TV, riding as a passenger in a car or sitting quietly after a meal, get checked for sleep apnea. I had a good friend who died from sleep apnea. He was only 37. His wife sent the kids in to wake Daddy because he was sleeping too late. Daddy had already passed. It's real!

If your airway is restricted because of large tonsils, a narrow palate, or a tongue that falls back when you sleep, you may be needlessly suffering from some form of Sleep Disordered Breathing. Dentists are working with physicians to make oral devices that open the airway for a better night's sleep. For some cases, a CPAP (Continuous Positive Airway Pressure) is best, but if the patient won't wear it, it's entirely ineffective. Oral devices may be an option.

A note on oral device alternative to CPAP

All dental sleep devices are Mandibular Advancement Devices (MAD). There are different designs, but all of them bring the mandible (lower jaw) forward, which opens the airway behind the tongue. Inquire with your dentist if you would like to try one. A MAD device should be provided through a qualified dentist who will have it custom-made for you.

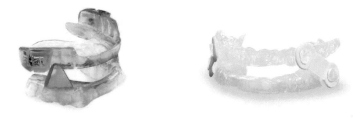

First, sleep studies are completed, either at your home or at a sleep lab, to determine if you have sleep apnea and how advanced it is. Once it's determined you're a candidate for an Oral Sleep Device, the dentist makes impressions of your teeth and measures your bite. Then, the dentist writes a prescription for the laboratory for fabrication. Once fabricated, the dentist fits the device, making sure the patient's jaw position is correct and that the appliance doesn't produce soreness in the mouth. Some devices can be found over the counter, but I don't recommend them. If the device fails to place the jaw in the right position, other problems can ensue such as TMJ, muscle soreness, and sometimes headaches.

Dry Mouth

Certain medications can negatively impact the health of your mouth. One common side effect is called *xerostomia*, a technical term for "dry mouth." A dry mouth lacks enough saliva to dilute the acid produced by the bacterial plaque on and between your teeth, and under your gums. The aging, accumulated plaque increases your cavity rate and worsens gum disease. Be sure to inform the dentist of any medications you're taking and if you've experienced dry mouth as a side effect.

In cases when you cannot stop the medication, your excellent homecare will empower you to avoid this damage to your mouth, the front door of your body.

Your Bite!

Hopefully, your bite is perfect. But if it's not, thankfully, checking your bite is more advanced today than it once was. In addition to articulating ribbon, that blue or red paper the dentist has you bite, there are thin, pressure-sensitive computer wafers that show where you touch when you bite, how hard you hit each spot, and the sequence in which your teeth touch. TekScan is one such device. Many times, it's your bite that is causing you headaches or tooth pain. Digitalized bite analysis helps identify where and when your teeth touch. Adjusting your bite can eliminate the pain. You can't treat what you can't find, but these new technologies can help you find (and repair) a bad bite.

These are the basic components of a complete dental examination. Be sure your dentist is thorough. Just like some physicians are more thorough than others, some dentists go deeper. It's about much more than your teeth. It could be your life. If you can find a dentist who includes at least these procedures in your oral exam, you're on the path to a healthy mouth.

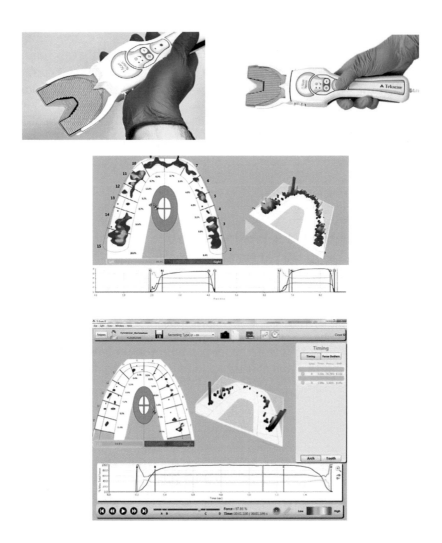

Consultation

Once the examination is completed and the dentist reviews the information, the dentist goes over the findings with you and presents treatment options. This is the consultation portion of your examination, which sometimes occurs during your first visit and other times at a subsequent appointment as needed. If your consultation seems overwhelming, please remember there are always options. Chapter 10 talks about the choices you have in your dental treatment. Not everyone drives a Lexus, but everybody needs transportation. Whichever options you choose, you can't let disease fester under your hood!

Getting past the Jitters to the Chair

A lot of people have had awkward or just plain bad experiences with dentists and, as a result, are nervous about ever sitting in the dentist's chair again. Unfortunately, as we saw with my patient's brother-in-law, never going back to the dental chair is not a good solution. If a previous bad experience has you anxious about going, there are a few things you can do.

For instance, some dentists provide sedation. If opting for sedation makes you feel better and less anxious about your upcoming dental treatment, talk with your dentist and plan on it in advance. The reassurance alone will make you feel better even before you get to the office. You will, however, need a driver for your dental appointment if you use sedation (which might be a bonus, as having someone with you there whom you trust already could ease your anxiety as well).

Another option is frequent short visits. Rather than starting with long procedures, begin with shorter, easier visits. Nothing builds confidence like success, and when you have successful, comfortable shorter visits, you can move to longer visits without the emotional stress.

I know someone who uses a few drops of essential oils to help her keep calm, and that works for her. Others take anti-anxiety medication. Use whatever support you need to keep calm and get yourself to the dentist. Your life and health truly depend on it. Most likely, after a few good dental visits, you'll no longer need the anxiety support. New experiences can replace old memories, but if you stop seeing the dentist for a while, your anxiety usually returns. So don't stop!

Let's review what we've learned so far:

1. The mouth is the front door to the body. Most bacteria enter the body through the front door. These bacteria cause or affect many medical problems: cardiovascular disease, heart attacks, strokes, E.D., diabetic and pregnancy complications, pneumonia, Alzheimer's disease, and rheumatoid arthritis. Lack of pain does not mean the mouth is healthy.

2. Most physicians were not trained to include the mouth as a part of a "complete" examination, but you can. You can bridge that deadly gap by choosing to have your mouth examined by a skilled dentist and then sharing the results of the oral exam with your physician. (We'll discuss how to share this information in Chapter 12).

3. Ask your doctor(s) "Does the health of my mouth have anything to do with the health of the rest of my body?" You already know the answer. You want to see what your doctor believes.

4. "Why" do I want a healthy mouth? Save money? Help prevent heart attacks, strokes, or other medical issues? Live longer? Know your why! Tape a motivating picture, photo, or money to your bathroom mirror.

5. It isn't sugar that causes cavities and gum disease. It's bacteria eating the sugar dumping acid on the teeth and gums. Decreasing sugar, thoroughly removing dental plaque (bacteria), and adding an oral probiotic are the keys.

6. How to clean your teeth involves removing the bacteria from the teeth without damaging the tooth or the gum. Tools: toothbrush, electric toothbrush, floss, interdental brushes, Directed Water Irrigation, Disclosing Tablets or Solution. Take 8-10 minutes one time a day.

7. Find the age-appropriate motivating factors. Sugar Bugs, sex appeal, or health. What do they "Want" or "Don't Want"?

8. Finding the right dentist for you and your family may take some work. You may have to visit several dentists before you find the dentist you are comfortable with and trust. The money you spend on finding the right dentist is money well spent.

9. A Complete Dental Examination includes but is not limited to medical, dental, and a medication history review, checking blood pressure and pulse, X-rays (single, bitewing, panoramic, and/or CBCT), photographs, periodontal probing, tooth by tooth examination, bite evaluation, oral cancer examination, sleep apnea evaluation, possibly saliva testing, and consultation with options for treatment.

Chapter 10

What Are My Options for Dental Treatment?

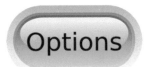

There are some real basics in dentistry. You only have so many choices, so let's start with the goal. First and most importantly, eliminate all infections in the teeth and gums. Once the infections are gone, it's a matter of being able to talk, chew, and smile.

You don't need teeth to have a healthy mouth, but if you have teeth, you can't allow infections. I would much rather see someone with no teeth than infected teeth. The infection doesn't stay in your mouth. It goes into your bloodstream and travels everywhere you have a blood supply. It may be undesirable, but if the situation becomes bad enough, the final option is to remove all your teeth and replace them with complete dentures or false teeth.

Your gums and bone are the foundation for your teeth. Lose the foundation—lose the teeth.

If you have gum disease (gingivitis or periodontitis), early treatment usually starts with cleaning your teeth. There are different levels of cleaning. If your gums bleed when you brush or floss, that's an early sign of gum disease. If your gums are generally healthy and you have some stain or light tartar (calculus) on your teeth, usually prophylaxis or a regular cleaning appointment is recommended. If you have inflammation or bone loss, you usually need a deeper cleaning.

"I just want my free cleaning!"

Some people tell the dentist they only want the "free" cleaning their insurance covers. The dentist can't do that. When the dentist puts in the code to send to the insurance company for regular cleaning (DN 1110), they are telling the insurance company you have a healthy mouth, no disease, and only need prophylaxis (regular cleaning). If you do have gum disease, the dentist has just lied to the insurance company and can face legal issues. Please don't ask the dentist to lie for you.

Deep cleanings do not have to be painful!

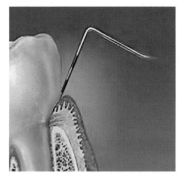 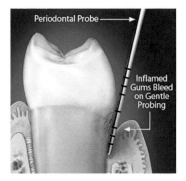

You can be numbed, so there isn't any pain. A deep cleaning might be your first step toward complete oral health.

Cleaning the part of your teeth that shows when you smile doesn't remove the bacteria and calculus (tartar) under your gums. Even with clean-looking teeth, gum disease will continue destroying the bone around your teeth and dumping harmful bacteria into your bloodstream. A regular cleaning won't stop the disease under the gum.

Depending on the severity of your gum disease, the dentist may recommend dental office hygiene visits every three, four, or six months. It all depends on your body's response and how thoroughly you clean your teeth at home.

Once the dentist or hygienist has helped you thoroughly clean your teeth, which might take several visits, you'll be able to maintain your teeth from home. As long as you keep up daily home maintenance, you should never need a deep cleaning again. Review Chapter 6 ("How to Thoroughly Clean Your Teeth") for simple and effective homecare instructions.

Gum Surgery

Gum surgery may be recommended, but typically only after you've exhausted all options to help the gums heal properly without surgery. Regardless, **if you're not willing to maintain your teeth at home, don't waste your money on gum surgery.** It won't work. You'll be throwing your money away and the gum disease will return.

What you do at home will make or break your gums. A thorough cleaning of 8-10 minutes daily will save you not only thousands of dollars but cut down the harmful bacteria flowing into your bloodstream.

"My teeth have problems. What are my options?"

What about repairing teeth? What methods are available to fix cavities, repair broken teeth, or replace missing teeth?

There are only so many options:

• Fillings

• Crowns

• Bridges

• Root Canals

• Extractions

• Implants

• Partial Dentures

• Complete Dentures

Fillings

Fillings do just what the word sounds like—fill in a tooth.

If you have a cavity but don't address it because there's no pain, the cavity will continue to grow until it hits the pulp (nerve) and causes a tooth abscess. This leaves you with no other choice but to get a root canal or an extraction. Don't wait. Fillings remove decay and restore a tooth to its original shape; thus, eliminating further risk to the tooth or gums.

Sometimes we'll place very large fillings to get tooth decay under control. Once the decay is under control, your dentist can go back at a later date and place crowns for strength where needed.

Most fillings today are Tooth-Colored Composite Restorations. Although amalgam (silver) fillings were very popular in the past, we have better materials today. People did not like that amalgam fillings turned black over time. Composite fillings, properly placed, blend in with the color of the natural teeth and can last for decades when maintained.

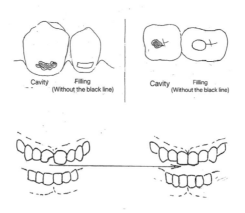

Fillings

Crowns (Caps)

When the cavity is large or the tooth is broken, you can still place a filling, but it may not be strong enough. Remember, a filling is meant to "fill in" a tooth. It was not designed to build a whole tooth. A stronger, more viable option would be a crown.

A crown (cap) covers the entire tooth and is much stronger than a filling. It generally takes two visits to complete. During the first visit, the dentist numbs the tooth, removes decay, shapes the tooth, and makes an impression of the prepared tooth either with impression material or digital images. With the physical or digital model of your prepared tooth, the dental laboratory can make a crown that fits well, looks great, and restores your tooth to its original color and shape. In the meantime, the dentist or assistant will make a temporary crown so you can smile and chew until the final crown is ready.

During your second visit, the dentist or assistant will remove the temporary crown and fit the final crown to your bite and to the teeth beside it. You need to be able to floss. If the contact is too tight, the floss frays. If it's too loose, food gets trapped. The dentist or assistant will hand you a mirror for your approval of the appearance. Once you approve, the dentist cements the cap onto your prepared tooth, lets it harden, and removes any excess cement. Usually, you are numbed both to prepare the tooth and cement the crown, although many people do not need to be numbed when cementing because there is no further drilling on the tooth. In this case, the numbing is only to help you feel more comfortable if that's helpful to you.

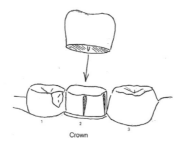

Crown

Crown, Covers the entire crown of the tooth.

Root Canals: They Don't Have to Hurt!

Removing as much decay as possible is always the goal. Sometimes decay grows right to the edge of the nerve. There are medications the dentist can place that will help heal the nerve. In the past, dentists would place calcium hydroxide. Today, there are more materials including Silver Diamide Fluoride (SDF), which kills cavity-causing bacteria without killing the nerve. Unfortunately, SDF turns that area of the tooth black. A white filling can be placed over the blackened tooth structure.

There is no guarantee that when decay is deep, removing the decay and placing medications will prevent a root canal, but it's certainly worth a try. If that fails, then you're looking at a root canal or an extraction.

Root canal treatment is one of those procedures you must do after carefully selecting a trusted dentist. The canal is a hollow tunnel through the root that houses the tooth's nerve and blood vessels. Root canal treatment first cleans and then seals the tunnel with an inert filling material like Gutta Percha. You want it done right the first time by a dentist or specialist (endodontist) who will get the tooth completely sealed. There will be no space left where bacteria can live and infect your bloodstream *if* the canal is sealed to the tip of the tooth. If not, the root canal will have to be re-treated until the tooth is fully sealed.

Root canals earned a bad reputation in the past because, many times, dentists worked on the tooth while it was still infected. It's very difficult to get a tooth numb where there is an active infection. Working on the infected tooth caused a lot of pain. Thankfully, it doesn't have to be that way anymore.

Today, the general process begins with getting the tooth infection under control using antibiotics. Once the infection is handled, it's much easier to get the tooth totally numb. Then, the dentist or specialist can comfortably enter the tooth and remove the infected nerve, blood vessels, and other debris from the canal.

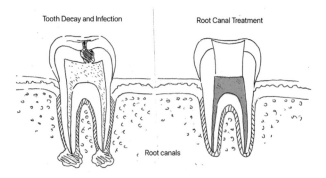

Tooth Decay and Infection   Root Canal Treatment

Root canals

Do I really need a crown after my root canal?

Once the root canal is done, the blood supply no longer flows to the treated tooth. The tooth then becomes brittle and breaks more easily. A crown is placed to fortify the tooth. If more support is needed, a "post" adds strength. In my career, I've seen hundreds of teeth that eventually broke and needed to be extracted because the patient went without a crown following root canals. It was a waste of the patient's time and money. If you're planning to get a root canal treatment, plan to get a crown if the dentist recommends one.

How can I replace missing teeth?

Suppose you lost a tooth due to decay, trauma, or that tooth was always missing (congenital). There are three options to replace it:

1. Removable Partial Denture: This is an appliance that you can easily insert and remove from your mouth. It hooks on to other teeth in that arch, fills in the space, keeps the other teeth from shifting around, and helps you chew. It's not as nice as your natural teeth, but it's better than having a mouthful of gaps, letting your teeth shift, changing your bite, and causing Temporo Mandibular Joint (TMJ) trauma or other issues. Both partial and complete dentures can accumulate tartar, not only making them smelly but also changing the shape so they don't fit correctly. To prevent this, you remove the partial denture at night just like your glasses and shoes. Regularly brush the partial denture to keep it clean. If you soak your partial or denture in white vinegar for 30 minutes, (not overnight) the tartar easily brushes off. This nighttime removal also allows your gum tissues time to rest.

Removable partial denture showing clasps (wires that go around teeth)

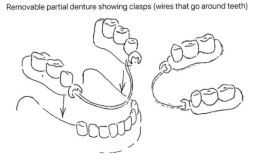

Removable partial denture replaces missing teeth and hooks on to remaining teeth

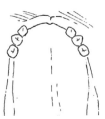
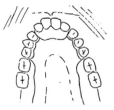

2. Fixed Bridge: A three-unit bridge is two crowns with a fake tooth in the middle to replace a single missing tooth. A bridge can also replace several teeth as long as the remaining teeth have adequate support. If you have solid teeth on either side of a missing tooth, you can usually place a fixed bridge. This involves doing crown preparations on the teeth next to the missing tooth and then fabricating the bridge. The teeth then become one solid piece. Cleaning is now more challenging because you can't get floss in between them. Therefore, using a floss threader, proxy brushes, or directed water irrigation (DWI) will clean the area nicely. I've had patients with bridges that have been in their mouth for over 40 years and are still going strong!

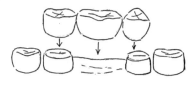

Dental Bridge: Replaces missing tooth.

3. Implants: An implant is a titanium screw that goes into the bone. It acts like the root of a tooth, *not* the entire tooth. It generally takes 3-4 months for the bone and titanium implant to "osteo-integrate," i.e. fuse together. Once they have osteo-integrated, you can place the crown. That happens in two steps. First, an *abutment* is made that screws into the implant. Then, a crown is placed over the abutment. The implant crown is similar to a natural tooth since you can brush, floss, chew, and smile with it. Although you will never get a cavity on an implant, you can still get gum disease—a leading cause of implant failure. You still have to keep it clean!

Single Implant

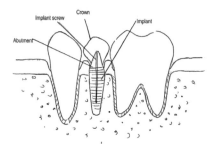

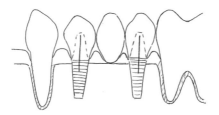

What if I'm going to lose all my teeth?

Most people do not like to walk around without teeth. Following extractions, you can opt for "immediate" denture placement. The immediate denture replaces the missing teeth while your gums and bone heal. This generally takes 2-3 months or longer. The immediate dentures will have to be adjusted as the gums heal. When all the extraction sites are healed and the gum is healthy, it's time to make the new final dentures or reline the immediate denture to the new shape of the gums. When you make new final dentures, you can use the immediate denture as a spare, just in case something happens to the final denture.

Getting used to dentures

Complete dentures are comparable to a prosthetic leg. People with prosthetic legs can learn to walk again. They just have to walk differently. It takes practice. The day you get the artificial leg is not the day you go on a long walk. There's a learning curve.

The upper denture is usually an easier adjustment than the lower. The roof of your mouth is called a palate. Your palate helps create a suction, which helps keep the upper denture in place. The lower denture has to deal with a tongue that knocks the denture loose when you talk. You must learn how to talk and chew all over again. It's not easy at first, but I've yet to see someone fail given a little patience and practice.

Years ago, I was at a water park in Central Florida with my kids. There was a young man there who had lost his leg above the knee. He was in front of us as we climbed up a long stairway to get to the top of a waterslide. This guy didn't miss a thing. Not only did he go down every slide in the park, but he did it at the same pace or faster than people with two healthy legs.

I guarantee you, this man wasn't so skilled with his prosthetic the first day he got it. It took practice and time. Complete dentures take practice, too.

Two hints I give to every complete denture patient:

1. Chew like an alligator, not like a cow. Chew straight up and down. If you move your jaw in a circular motion, you'll knock the denture loose.

2. You cannot have a favorite side. You must have food on both sides (left and right). Then, chew straight up and down. If you chew on one side, the denture will usually pop loose on the other side. If you chew on both sides, it's easier to keep the denture in place.

It generally takes about a month for people to learn how to chew with complete dentures.

Note: Denture adhesives help to keep the dentures in place and are available at most grocery stores or pharmacies. Keep in mind that adhesives may loosen throughout the day and need to be reapplied.

Complete dentures

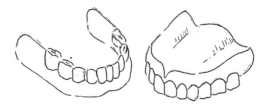

"My dentures are loose and I don't like denture adhesives."

If you still have problems, you still have options. If your dentures are loose, many times you can re-line the dentures to the new shape of your gums and bone. Our body changes shape throughout our lives. That includes the mouth and jaw bones. The relined dentures may solve your looseness problem. You'll probably need adjustments after the reline, just like a new denture.

You can also place implants into the bone, then snap the removable complete denture onto the implants. This is especially helpful for a lower denture.

You still remove and clean the dentures nightly, which, again, gives your gum tissue a rest.

Implant Supported Denture

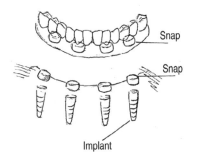
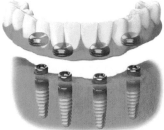

Choose Wisely

We've now covered the basic options for your dental treatment. Keeping your original teeth clean and healthy is our first goal. When life happens and we have to compromise, review your options before deciding on treatment.

You can't un-ring a bell. All decisions have consequences, either good or bad. The consequences of bad teeth can be life-changing and sometimes life-ending. The consequences of good teeth are better health, enjoying your smile, and enjoying every meal. Some people believe we came to earth for the food. If so, let's enjoy every bite!

Let's review what we've learned so far:

1. The mouth is the front door to the body. Most bacteria enter the body through the front door. These bacteria cause or affect many medical problems: cardiovascular disease, heart attacks, strokes, E.D., diabetic and pregnancy complications, pneumonia, Alzheimer's disease, and rheumatoid arthritis. Lack of pain does not mean the mouth is healthy.

2. Most physicians were not trained to include the mouth as a part of a "complete" examination, but you can. You can bridge that deadly gap by choosing to have your mouth examined by a skilled dentist and then sharing the results of the oral exam with your physician. (We'll discuss how to share this information in Chapter 12).

3. Ask your doctor(s) "Does the health of my mouth have anything to do with the health of the rest of my body?" You already know the answer. You want to see what your doctor believes.

4. "Why" do I want a healthy mouth? Save money? Help prevent heart attacks, strokes, or other medical issues? Live longer? Know your why! Tape a motivating picture, photo, or money to your bathroom mirror.

5. It isn't sugar that causes cavities and gum disease. It's bacteria eating the sugar dumping acid on the teeth and gums. Decreasing sugar, thoroughly removing dental plaque (bacteria), and adding an oral probiotic are the keys.

6. How to clean your teeth involves removing the bacteria from the teeth without damaging the tooth or the gum. Tools: toothbrush, electric toothbrush, floss, interdental brushes, Directed Water Irrigation, Disclosing Tablets or Solution. Take 8-10 minutes one time a day.

7. Find the age-appropriate motivating factors. Sugar Bugs, sex appeal, or health. What do they "Want" or "Don't Want"?

8. Finding the right dentist for you and your family may take some work. You may have to visit several dentists before you find the dentist you are comfortable with and trust. The money you spend on finding the right dentist is money well spent.

9. A Complete Dental Examination includes but is not limited to medical, dental, and a medication history review, checking blood pressure and pulse, X-rays (single, bitewing, panoramic, and/or CBCT), photographs, periodontal probing, tooth by tooth examination, bite evaluation, oral cancer examination, sleep apnea evaluation, possibly saliva testing, and consultation with options for treatment.

10. There are numerous treatment options. Removing all infection is the first step, followed by removing decay, restoring teeth, replacing missing teeth, and daily maintenance (8-10 minutes).

Chapter 11

Begin at Home Today
It's Critical and It's <u>FREE</u>

If you're getting snagged on finances or schedules, or you just don't like going to the dentist, I have good news for you. Excellent oral care begins at home, usually in the bathroom by the sink in front of a mirror.

Review Chapter 6 on "How to Thoroughly Clean Your Teeth." What you do at your sink could save time, money, and health—or *cost* you time, money, and health. Disease does not get the final say. You have power. You have a choice! Right there in a simple toothbrush and some thread (floss), you have the power to begin transforming your health and make a long, healthy life more than possible—maybe even predictable.

The Right Environment

You can't control everything that happens in life, but you can control your home environment enough to either support or hinder your goals. Create a space that makes it easy to practice your new healthy habits.

Perhaps you've already placed your "why" where you will see it, such as taped to the bathroom mirror where you brush. So that you're not relying on motivation alone, do some planning. If you keep your floss tucked away inside a medicine cabinet that you never open, you'll only get to it when you "feel" like it, if then. Instead, put your electric toothbrush, toothpaste, floss, and any other oral care tools where you'll be most likely to see—and use—them every day.

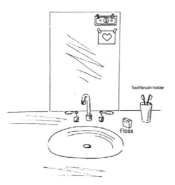

If the dentist cleans your teeth and fills your cavities, but you go home and never do daily homecare, your dentist's work will fail. The cavities will come back. Oral bacteria will continue dumping acid onto your teeth resulting in new cavities or cavities next to your new fillings. The gums will become infected and bleed, dumping bacteria back into your bloodstream, increasing the risk for heart attack, stroke, and other medical issues. You will have wasted your time and money.

Start your healthy mouth journey at home.

The $25 Oral Care Budget

You can begin today. It doesn't take much money or time. Brushing and flossing are free after the initial investment, and how much time do you spend on your phone? It's probably more than 8-10 minutes a day. Instead of watching that next YouTube video, pause it and give yourself the oral care that you deserve. While you're at it, throw on some relaxing music to accompany you as you do your routine. The benefits of your relaxation and self-care will far outweigh the sacrifice of a few minutes. In the long run, taking care of your mouth will save you thousands of dollars in dental treatments and help avoid many medical problems. It's always worth it every single day.

About $25-$30 and 8-10 minutes daily are all you need. You can always spend more, but let's start with the basics:

1. A good, soft toothbrush: $5-7

2. Toothpaste (non-abrasive): $2-$5

3. Floss (whatever floss works better for you): $5 or less

4. Disclosing Solution (drug store or online): $10-$15

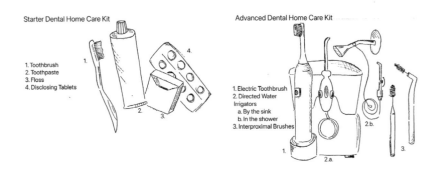

Starter Dental Home Care Kit
1. Toothbrush
2. Toothpaste
3. Floss
4. Disclosing Tablets

Advanced Dental Home Care Kit
1. Electric Toothbrush
2. Directed Water Irrigators
  a. By the sink
  b. In the shower
3. Interproximal Brushes

Behind the Curtain of Your Lips

If we removed your lips and cheeks so you could look directly at your teeth and gums, many people would be shocked to discover cavities that *look* painful, but which were hiding there silently and painlessly. The gums are often red, swollen, and bleed easily.

How often should we clean a wound? Every day! We must clean our oral wounds if we expect them to get better instead of worse. Dirty wounds release more pus into the bloodstream. That's not healthy.

Here's the Sequence for Cleaning:

1. Brush, floss, water irrigate, proxy brush, etc.

2. Chew a disclosing tablet or rinse disclosing solution. Rinse with water. Then check to see any remaining plaque.

3. Examine and grade your thoroughness (be honest—there are no consequences for struggling while learning these habits, but there are consequences for doing an incomplete job).

4. Remove the remaining plaque shown by the disclosing solution.

5. Repeat as necessary.

At first, disclose once per week. As your home cleanings become more efficient, once per month will be sufficient. Just be sure and check. It may feel emotionally good to avoid looking but incurring preventable damage because of failure to check will ultimately feel bad—physically, emotionally, and financially. It's always better to know for sure.

When Homecare Is Not Enough

You can start the dental health process without a dentist, but you'll need one to help you finish.

There are some infections you can't clean out with a toothbrush or floss. Sometimes, severely infected teeth must be removed; cavities must be cleaned out and filled; calculus (tartar) on your teeth is too stubborn for your toothbrush and will need to be professionally removed. Keep in mind that numbing and sedation are always available.

Healthy mouths don't pollute the bloodstream with harmful pathogens. Having no gum disease or cavities is the goal. Start the process of achieving good oral health today beginning with the affordable stuff that you can do on your own. Get your toothbrush and floss ready for use. Keep them where you can get to them easily. Follow the steps. Trust the process. Start getting completely dentally healthy today. Your body will thank you.

Let's review what we've learned so far:

1. The mouth is the front door to the body. Most bacteria enter the body through the front door. These bacteria cause or affect many medical problems: cardiovascular disease, heart attacks, strokes, E.D., diabetic and pregnancy complications, pneumonia, Alzheimer's disease, and rheumatoid arthritis. Lack of pain does not mean the mouth is healthy.

2. Most physicians were not trained to include the mouth as a part of a "complete" examination, but you can. You can bridge that deadly gap by choosing to have your mouth examined by a skilled dentist and then sharing the results of the oral exam with your physician. (We'll discuss how to share this information in Chapter 12).

3. Ask your doctor(s) "Does the health of my mouth have anything to do with the health of the rest of my body?" You already know the answer. You want to see what your doctor believes.

4. "Why" do I want a healthy mouth? Save money? Help prevent heart attacks, strokes, or other medical issues? Live longer? Know your why! Tape a motivating picture, photo, or money to your bathroom mirror.

5. It isn't sugar that causes cavities and gum disease. It's bacteria eating the sugar dumping acid on the teeth and gums. Decreasing sugar, thoroughly removing dental plaque (bacteria), and adding an oral probiotic are the keys.

6. How to clean your teeth involves removing the bacteria from the teeth without damaging the tooth or the gum. Tools: toothbrush, electric toothbrush, floss, interdental brushes, Directed Water Irrigation, Disclosing Tablets or Solution. Take 8-10 minutes one time a day.

7. Find the age-appropriate motivating factors. Sugar Bugs, sex appeal, or health. What do they "Want" or "Don't Want"?

8. Finding the right dentist for you and your family may take some work. You may have to visit several dentists before you find the dentist you are comfortable with and trust. The money you spend on finding the right dentist is money well spent.

9. A Complete Dental Examination includes but is not limited to medical, dental, and a medication history review, checking blood pressure and pulse, X-rays (single, bitewing, panoramic, and/or CBCT), photographs, periodontal probing, tooth by tooth examination, bite evaluation, oral cancer examination, sleep apnea evaluation, possibly saliva testing, and consultation with options for treatment.

10. There are numerous treatment options. Removing all infection is the first step, followed by removing decay, restoring teeth, replacing missing teeth, and daily maintenance (8-10 minutes).

11. You can begin your journey to a healthy mouth even before you see a dentist. The tools needed are inexpensive. The biggest investment is in your time and effort. You will probably need a dentist to help you complete your journey.

Chapter 12

End the Deadly Gap
Start the Communication

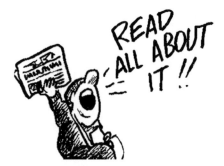

You Didn't Know What You Didn't Know

You now know more about the oral-systemic connection than many doctors! It's sad but true that neither you nor your friends were ever likely to get this information from medical professionals. Often, it's not even their fault. As we now know, most doctors' training lacked any emphasis on the importance of the connection between your mouth and your body.

The truth about your mouth must spread by word of mouth—pun definitely intended! The mouth is a part of the body as vital to your overall health as any other part. If the goal is the patient's health, physicians must begin to include the mouth when diagnosing and treating illnesses.

Poor diet and lack of adequate oral hygiene in the United States have increased the incidence of dental disease. Poorer countries with less sugar in their diet have fewer dental issues. The Standard American Diet (SAD) is unlike that of many countries. It fuels oral bacteria. It is high in sugar and carbohydrates, which leads to higher percentages of the population having cavities and gum disease. Oral bacteria are silently damaging the health of millions of people in the United States right now. As you share what you've learned here, you can help change that.

Do Your Own Research

It's good to do your own research, so I've provided many links to published research at the end of this book. Learn how dental bacteria affect cardiovascular disease, and which oral bacteria researchers are discovering in the brains of Alzheimer's patients. See what it does to diabetes. Look at the statistics. The mouth is the biggest polluter of the body!

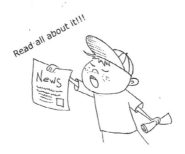

Who is Responsible?

Who is going to tell your mom and dad? Who is going to tell your children, or your brothers and sisters? Who is going to help them understand how dental bacteria affects their heart or diabetes or pregnancy?

Over 600,000 people die each year in the United States from heart attacks. Roughly 50% of heart attacks are triggered by dental infections. **That means over 300,000 people in the United States die each year from heart attacks triggered by preventable oral infections.** This doesn't even include those who survived but now have new heart valves, stents, a lifetime of medications, and much more. We've already covered why physicians, dentists, and other healthcare providers aren't telling you. They weren't trained to tell you.

Who should tell our families about how much dental health affects our overall health? Who will tell your friends and coworkers? If not you, who?

Share with Family & Friends

Sharing this book might be the quickest way to help others understand the importance of their dental health. Loan it to them. Give it to them. Buy them an extra book to give to someone else. **All profits from the sale of this book will go to The Dental Medical Convergence, Inc., a 501c3 non-profit with the mission of educating families and healthcare professionals about the oral-systemic connection** (visit them at www.TheDentalMedicalConvergence.org). If you have the means, you could buy the books in bulk to share with your local clinics, schools, church, or book club.

When you help others connect the dots between their dental health and their heart, pancreas, brain, lungs, and whole body, you potentially save their lives. Armed with simple instructions to properly clean their teeth, they will remember YOU for helping them save time, energy, and major expenses, not to mention the pain, suffering, and loss of life that may result from otherwise preventable illness.

You *can* control your dental expenses and so can everyone around you. To do that, they must be told the truth and, just like you, they have to want it for themselves. It's not selfish to take care of yourself first and *then* encourage others to do the same. In fact, it's the opposite of selfish because the healthier you are, the less burdensome you are to others, and the more you can help when you find others in need. As much as needed, go back to Chapters 6 and 11 to review homecare methods so you can stay on track and healthy. Let your own glowing health inspire others as you share all that you've learned in this book and through your own routine.

Share with Dentists & Physicians

As a dentist, I found that when patients understood what I've shared with you in this book, their willingness and ability to "comply" with my recommendations dramatically improved. Share this book with your dentists and physicians, and you'll be helping to ease a common source of frustration for dental and medical professionals—when our patients suffer needlessly for simply refusing to do what we recommend. I expect that when your dentist shares the information, they'll enjoy the same success with their patients.

Good dentists want their patients' mouths to be healthy and disease-free. Don't worry about dentists keeping busy. There is plenty of restorative and replacement work to keep dentists in business for the rest of their lives. Once your dentists and physicians see how motivated their patients become when armed with this simple, life-changing information, they will use it, and they will thank you.

Share to Solve Medical Riddles

Reading this book may also help your doctor solve years-long riddles as they discover some patients' "incurable" conditions were actually caused by poor oral health all along, and may also be improved or cleared completely by treating the patient's mouth. Many fantastic physicians just want the best for their patients. They think about them at night, trying to figure out the source of bacteria and disease. They simply have yet to connect the dots between dental disease and the rest of the body. Urge your physician to include your mouth as a component of medical and physical examinations. Hand them a copy (or ten) of this book. A truly good physician whose priority is your health will not be offended by this.

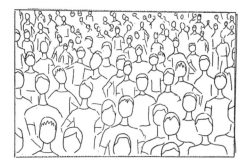

"Don't Ask, Don't Tell" Doesn't Work

Ninety percent of dental infections have no pain. Patients don't know. Doctors don't ask. Dentists don't tell. It's a losing combination. Let's change it!

There must be dialogue between physicians and dentists. It's the same body, the same blood, the same person we're both serving. When we work together, everybody wins.

Hopefully, you now understand the importance of your oral health and you are ready to take action. If your mouth is in great shape today, you know how to maintain it. If it needs work, you know the steps to fix it.

Know your *why*. Grab your supplies. Start with your tiny habit. High-five yourself in the mirror on the way out.

And know that you're now a positive force in the world who's helping to close *the deadly gap*.

Let's review what we've learned so far:

1. The mouth is the front door to the body. Most bacteria enter the body through the front door. These bacteria cause or affect many medical problems: cardiovascular disease, heart attacks, strokes, E.D., diabetic and pregnancy complications, pneumonia, Alzheimer's disease, and rheumatoid arthritis. Lack of pain does not mean the mouth is healthy.

2. Most physicians were not trained to include the mouth as a part of a "complete" examination, but you can. You can bridge that deadly gap by choosing to have your mouth examined by a skilled dentist and then sharing the results of the oral exam with your physician. (We'll discuss how to share this information in Chapter 12).

3. Ask your doctor(s) "Does the health of my mouth have anything to do with the health of the rest of my body?" You already know the answer. You want to see what your doctor believes.

4. "Why" do I want a healthy mouth? Save money? Help prevent heart attacks, strokes, or other medical issues? Live longer? Know your why! Tape a motivating picture, photo, or money to your bathroom mirror.

5. It isn't sugar that causes cavities and gum disease. It's bacteria eating the sugar dumping acid on the teeth and gums. Decreasing sugar, thoroughly removing dental plaque (bacteria), and adding an oral probiotic are the keys.

6. How to clean your teeth involves removing the bacteria from the teeth without damaging the tooth or the gum. Tools: toothbrush, electric toothbrush, floss, interdental brushes, Directed Water Irrigation, Disclosing Tablets or Solution. Take 8-10 minutes one time a day.

7. Find the age-appropriate motivating factors. Sugar Bugs, sex appeal, or health. What do they "Want" or "Don't Want"?

8. Finding the right dentist for you and your family may take some work. You may have to visit several dentists before you find the dentist you are comfortable with and trust. The money you spend on finding the right dentist is money well spent.

9. A Complete Dental Examination includes but is not limited to medical, dental, and a medication history review, checking blood pressure and pulse, X-rays (single, bitewing, panoramic, and/or CBCT), photographs, periodontal probing, tooth by tooth examination, bite evaluation, oral cancer examination, sleep apnea evaluation, possibly saliva testing, and consultation with options for treatment.

10. There are numerous treatment options. Removing all infection is the first step, followed by removing decay, restoring teeth, replacing missing teeth, and daily maintenance (8–10 minutes).

11. You can begin your journey to a healthy mouth even before you see a dentist. The tools needed are inexpensive. The biggest investment is in your time and effort. You will probably need a dentist to help you complete your journey.

12. Spread the word. Share with family, friends, dentists, and physicians. You could help improve the quality of life of friends and family or even save a life!

A PERSONAL NOTE

I wrote this book in hopes of helping you and your family stay healthier, avoid preventable medical issues, and save thousands of dollars in dental care. When you truly "get it" you can be an example for your family. It's absolutely amazing what 8-10 minutes a day can do for you!

In the interest of your better dental and medical health,

DR. CHUCK

REFERENCES SHOWING THE LINKS BETWEEN ORAL HEALTH AND OVERALL HEALTH:

(Please search online for additional research coming out regularly.)

GENERAL

Oral Health in America: A Report of the Surgeon General
https://www.nidcr.nih.gov/sites/default/files/2017-10/
hck1ocv.%40www.surgeon.fullrpt.pdf

The U.S Surgeon General's Report on Oral Health Executive Summary (July 2000)
https://www.nidcr.nih.gov/research/data-statistics/surgeon-general

2020 Surgeon General's Report: Oral Health in America: Advances and Challenges
https://www.nidcr.nih.gov/sites/default/files/2020-02/Surgeon-Generals-Report-2020_APHA3_Nov_2019_508_0.pdf

ScienceDirect: Oral infections and systemic disease—an emerging problem in medicine
https://www.sciencedirect.com/science/article/pii/S1198743X14625623

Washington State Department of Health: Oral Diseases and Other Systemic Conditions
https://doh.wa.gov/sites/default/files/legacy/Documents/Pubs//160-001-OralDiseasesSystemic.pdf

American Society for Microbiology: Systemic Diseases Caused by Oral Infections
https://journals.asm.org/doi/10.1128/cmr.13.4.547

Mayo Clinic: Oral health: A window to your overall health
https://www.mayoclinic.org/healthy-lifestyle/adult-health/in-depth/dental/art-20047475

ENP Manifesto: Perio and General Health
https://thedentalmedicalconvergence.org/wp-content/uploads/2021/12/EFP_manifesto_full_version_2016.pdf

Oral health's inextricable connection to systemic health: Special populations bring to bear multimodal relationships and factors connecting periodontal disease to systemic diseases and conditions
https://onlinelibrary.wiley.com/doi/epdf/10.1111/prd.12398

The Stockholm Study: Over 30 years' Observation of the Effect of Oral Infections on Systemic Health
https://www.ncbi.nlm.nih.gov/pmc/articles/PMC9030271/

The vital importance of the oral systemic link
https://oralsystemiclink.net/health-care-providers

Baseline Oral Health Study: Uncover the connections to general health
https://www.clinicaltrials.gov/ct2/show/NCT04954313

CARDIOVASCULAR

Harvard Medical School: Gum disease and heart disease
https://www.health.harvard.edu/heart-health/gum-disease-and-heart-disease-the-common-thread

National Institutes of Health: The link between periodontal disease and cardiovascular disease
https://www.ncbi.nlm.nih.gov/pmc/articles/PMC3100856/

Journal of Periodontology: Role for Periodontal Bacteria in Cardiovascular Diseases
https://pubmed.ncbi.nlm.nih.gov/11887470/

Science Daily: Connection between mouth bacteria, inflammation in heart disease
https://www.sciencedaily.com/releases/2015/04/150416132205.htm

The BMJ Postgraduate Medical Journal: High-risk periodontal pathogens contribute to the pathogenesis of atherosclerosis
https://pmj.bmj.com/content/93/1098/215

Cleveland Clinic: Oral Health & Risk for CV Disease
https://my.clevelandclinic.org/health/articles/11264-oral-health--risk-for-cv-disease

HEART ATTACK

Can a Tooth Infection Cause A Heart Attack?
https://www.epainassist.com/chest-pain/heart/can-a-tooth-infection-cause-a-heart-attack

Dental infections as a risk factor for acute myocardial infarction
https://pubmed.ncbi.nlm.nih.gov/8131788/

STROKE

American Heart Association: Oral Bacterial Signatures in Cerebral Thrombi of Patients With Acute Ischemic Stroke Treated With Thrombectomy
https://www.ahajournals.org/doi/10.1161/JAHA.119.012330

Stroke: A Journal of Cerebral Circulation: Periodontal Disease as a Risk Factor for Ischemic Stroke
https://www.ahajournals.org/doi/full/10.1161/01.STR.0000110789.20526.9D

Medscape: More Evidence Links Gum Disease to Stroke Risk
https://www.medscape.com/viewarticle/891550

Saebo: The Hidden Connection Between Gum Disease and Stroke
https://www.saebo.com/blog/the-hidden-connection-between-gum-disease-and-stroke/

National Institutes for Health: Gingivitis and periodontitis as a risk factor for stroke: A case-control study in the Iranian population
https://www.ncbi.nlm.nih.gov/pmc/articles/PMC3858735/

PubMed: Association between periodontal disease and stroke
https://pubmed.ncbi.nlm.nih.gov/22244863/

How oral health may affect your heart, brain and risk of death
https://www.heart.org/en/news/2021/03/19/how-oral-health-may-affect-your-heart-brain-and-risk-of-death

Does Oral Health Affect Your Heart?
https://cdnapisec.kaltura.com/index.php/extwidget/preview/partner_id/2207941/uiconf_id/37292221/entry_id/1_ukq1ehcd/embed/dynamic

Poor oral health and blood pressure control among US hypertensive adults
https://www.ahajournals.org/doi/10.1161/HYPERTENSIONAHA.118.11528

DIABETES

National Institutes of Health: Periodontitis and diabetes: a two-way relationship
https://www.ncbi.nlm.nih.gov/pmc/articles/PMC3228943/

American Diabetes Association: Diabetes and Periodontal Infection: Making the Connection
https://diabetesjournals.org/clinical/article/23/4/171/1633/Diabetes-and-Periodontal-Infection-Making-the

Diabetes and Oral Health (CDC)
https://www.cdc.gov/diabetes/managing/diabetes-oral-health.html

Diabetes and Oral Health (American Diabetes Association)
https://diabetes.org/diabetes/keeping-your-mouth-healthy

Oral Health and Diabetes (PubMed)
https://pubmed.ncbi.nlm.nih.gov/33651538/

ALZHEIMER'S DISEASE

National Health Institute: Periodontitis and Alzheimer's Disease: A Possible Comorbidity between Oral Chronic Inflammatory Condition and Neuroinflammation
https://www.ncbi.nlm.nih.gov/pmc/articles/PMC5649154/

Science Daily: Link between gum disease and cognitive decline in Alzheimer's
https://www.sciencedaily.com/releases/2016/03/160310141330.htm

Science Alert: The cause of Alzheimer's could be coming from inside your mouth, study claims
https://www.sciencealert.com/new-evidence-reveals-an-unexpected-culprit-behind-alzheimer-s-disease

PREGNANCY

Oral health during pregnancy
https://www.aafp.org/pubs/afp/issues/2008/0415/p1139.html

ScienceDirect: Periodontal disease and pregnancy outcomes: exposure, risk and intervention
https://www.sciencedirect.com/science/article/abs/pii/S1521693407000065

Dentaid: Periodontal disease and pregnancy
https://www.slideshare.net/Dentaid/periodontal-disease-and-pregnancy

Medical Life Sciences News: Periodontitis and Pregnancy
https://www.news-medical.net/health/Periodontitis-and-Pregnancy.aspx

Victoria State Government (Australia): Pregnancy and teeth
https://www.betterhealth.vic.gov.au/health/healthyliving/pregnancy-and-teeth

ARTHRITIS

Biomed Central: The association between rheumatoid arthritis and periodontal disease
https://arthritis-research.biomedcentral.com/articles/10.1186/ar3106

Gum disease linked to rheumatoid arthritis
https://www.hopkinsrheumatology.org/2017/01/gum-disease-linked-to-rheumatoid-arthritis/

Everyday Health: Rheumatoid Arthritis and Gum Disease: What You Need to Know
https://www.everydayhealth.com/rheumatoid-arthritis/living-with/the-link-between-gum-disease-and-rheumatoid-arthritis/

National Institutes of Health: Periodontal disease and rheumatoid arthritis: the evidence accumulates for complex pathobiologic interactions
https://www.ncbi.nlm.nih.gov/pmc/articles/PMC4495574/

National Rheumatoid Arthritis Society (UK): Gum Disease
https://nras.org.uk/resource/gum-disease/

NBC News: Could Gum Disease Cause Rheumatoid Arthritis?
https://www.nbcnews.com/health/health-news/could-gum-disease-cause-rheumatoid-arthritis-n695941

Rheumatology Advisor: Bi-Directional Links Between Rheumatoid Arthritis and Periodontal Disease
https://www.rheumatologyadvisor.com/home/topics/rheumatoid-arthritis/bi-directional-links-between-rheumatoid-arthritis-and-periodontal-disease/

PNEUMONIA

Association between oral health and incidence of pneumonia: a population-based cohort study from Korea
https://www.nature.com/articles/s41598-020-66312-2

Pneumonia incidence and oral health management by dental hygienists in long-term care facilities: A 1-year prospective multicentre cohort study
https://pubmed.ncbi.nlm.nih.gov/34750855/

WHITE COAT SYNDROME

People with Untreated "White Coat Hypertension" Twice as Likely to Die from Heart Disease
https://www.pennmedicine.org/news/news-releases/2019/june/people-untreated-white-coat-hypertension-twice-likely-die-heart-disease